Advance Praise

As a therapist and an autistic myself, I witness each day that many obstacles in life decrease as the ability to implement executive function skills increase. Based on research and implementing evidence-based practices, this book practically guides the reader with specific strategies to support executive function development so meaningful life outcomes can be attained across the age span for autistics.

~ Judy Endow, LCSW, Autism educational consultant, clinical therapist, award winning author and international speaker

As an autistic adult and certified occupational therapy assistant, I found this book to contain some invaluable tools supporting executive functioning skills. It provides an efficient framework for structuring the partnership between teacher and student to promote success across the lifespan. I will be implementing many of these strategies, both personally and as a clinician, for years to come!

~ Kelly Londenberg, Certified Occupational Therapy Assistant (COTA)

Executive function (EF) skills such as time management, organization, planning, problem solving, and emotional regulation are often not emphasized during the school years in favor of an academic curriculum; yet without solid EF skills, a person will struggle in their workplace, community, home, and relationships. Authors Carol Burmeister, Sheri Wilkins, and Rebecca Silva embrace this topic with enthusiasm and experience, and impart practical strategies and tools that are visual and/or tactile to implement their FLIPP (EF) acronym.

Using evidence-based practices and data collection for assessment and evaluation for educators, the authors empower students to make choices from a variety of options that are right for them and can be implemented in practical and meaningful ways. Supporting greater independence and engagement are the underpinning of these options. The book is peppered with excellent visual examples such as charts, templates, and forms to provide guidance and attain these goals. Educators are given several ideas for teaching and application of each skill in order to tailor a program to their unique student.

FLIPP 2.0 is a book that can grow with students as they gain skills and move to higher and more complex stages of learning. These tools can follow students into adulthood to help them successfully manage their home and work life. Building an EF skills foundation during the school years is an important part of a person's well-being, therefore working on these skills is good for all students!

~ Maureen Bennie, Director, Autism Awareness Centre Inc.

Many times, books for teachers working with children with disabilities are theoretical and the information is difficult to apply in both the general education and special education classrooms. FLIPP 2.0 provides a connection between best practices and the classroom in every chapter. What is most powerful about FLIPP 2.0 is it provides a voice for the students, providing activities that embed self-advocacy skills, empowering the students to develop strong executive function skills.

This book is a must-have for teachers, school administrators, school psychologists, counselors, and behavior specialists. The lessons can be implemented by both credentialed staff as well as paraprofessionals as a part of the daily school routine as well as provide foundational strategies to support classroom management and academic instruction. FLIPP 2.0 will be built into our professional learning communities as a tool to build our teachers' understanding of executive function, as well as a data tool to measure student performance. The forms provided as part of the book will be the perfect tool to measure student progress and will be incorporated into student portfolios for work experience and community service projects.

~ Lisa Kistler, Director of Special Education, Beaumont Unified School District

The perfect follow-up to FLIPP the Switch, FLIPP 2.0 provides educators and parents guidance and resources to support the executive functioning needs of individuals with Autism Spectrum Disorder (ASD), both in and out of the classroom. The authors have shared their decades of expertise and real-life experiences in an easily accessible book. Classroom teachers are provided with information about evidence-based practices (EBPs) that can be utilized in the learning environment and specifically designed for students with ASD. The text is wonderfully designed to take the reader on a learning journey around how to leverage EBPs to support students with ASD to reach their full potential. Love, love the visual examples and step-by-step directions. Well done, my friends.

~ Jacque Williams, Assistant Superintendent, West San Gabriel Valley SELPA

In FLIPP 2.0, Burmeister, Wilkins, and Silva brilliantly combine the science of executive function deficits with evidence-based strategies that can be easily implemented in the classroom or in the home. Drawn from the authors' lived and professional experience and illustrated with examples, templates, and scripts, FLIPP 2.0 is an indispensable resource of practical and effective approaches to support the remediation of executive function skill deficits. This book is an absolute must-read for teachers and parents seeking strategies to help the child experience success for a lifetime.

~ Ronald J. Powell, Ph.D., President, RJ Powell Consultants; educator; coauthor of Guided Growth; Educational Interventions for Children and Teens with Fetal Alcohol Spectrum Disorders and Early Trauma

FLIPP 2.0 is filled with so many great strategies for treatment teams to be proactive in preventing problem behaviors for people on the autism spectrum. Executive functioning deficits are often a barrier in all learning settings, however the strategies in this book reduce these barriers and promote access to instruction. All of the strategies in this book can be targeted across learning environments, school, home, and clinic, and are easily implemented by teachers, parents, behavior analysts and the student themselves. This book is especially unique in providing a guide for young adults to initiate EF strategies that will allow them to set up supports and environments to promote success. This book is a great resource for teaching EF skills in a fun and practical way and valuable for me as a behavior analyst.

~ Ashlee Keuneke, MA, BCBA

FLIPP 2.0 provides a key piece of the puzzle in truly supporting student achievement and success. Educators must focus on the student as a whole and this book provides insight into a crucial component of how students learn. FLIPP 2.0 provides educators with the knowledge and understanding of how executive functioning impacts student learning and how teachers can support this area in daily classroom routines. Furthermore, FLIPP 2.0 illustrates a cohesive approach to teach executive functioning skills by explaining theoretical concepts that serve as a foundation to then create instruction that embeds the use of evidence-based practices in meaningful and engaging activities.

After reading the book, educators will possess practical strategies that can be immediately implemented in the classroom. This book can support students from early elementary to adulthood and give them tools that can be used for the rest of their lives. Overall, it is an engaging read that will serve as a support for educators, students, and families. A must-have for every educator!

~Gaby Toledo, Special Education Coordinator, Beaumont Unified School District

FLIPP 2.0:

Mastering Executive Function Skills from School to Adult Life for Students with Autism

Carol Burmeister, M.A.

Sheri Wilkins, Ph.D.

Rebecca Silva, Ph.D.

AAPC PUBLISHING
PO Box 861116
Shawnee, KS 66216

Local Phone (913) 897-1004 Fax (913) 728-6090
www.aapcautismbooks.com

Published April 2021 by AAPC Publishing

Names: Burmeister, Carol Ann, author. | Silva, Rebecca, author. | Wilkins, Sheri (Sheri Ann), author. | Myles, Brenda Smith, writer of foreword.
Title: FLIPP 2.0 : mastering executive function skills from school to adult life for students with autism / Carol Burmeister, Rebecca Silva, Sheri Wilkins ; foreword by Brenda Smith Myles.
Description: [Second edition]. | Shawnee, KS : AAPC Publishing, [2021] | Revision of Wilkins and Burmeister's "FLIPP the switch" (AAPC Publishing, 2015). | Includes bibliographical references and index.

Identifiers: ISBN: 978-1-942197-63-8 (paperback) | 978-1-942197-64-5 (ebook)
Subjects: LCSH: Executive ability in children. | Executive functions (Neuropsychology) | Children with autism spectrum disorders-- Counseling of. | Success in children. | Children--Life skills guides. | Academic achievement. | Attention in children. | Problem solving in children. | Adaptability (Psychology) in children. | Impulse control disorders in children. | Emotional maturity.

Classification: LCC: BF723.E93 W55 2021 | DDC: 155.4/13--dc23

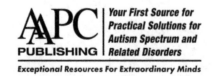

AAPC PUBLISHING — Your First Source for Practical Solutions for Autism Spectrum and Related Disorders

Exceptional Resources For Extraordinary Minds

Dedication

This book is dedicated to the students and families affected by autism whom we have had the pleasure to support over the years. *FLIPP 2.0* would never have been possible had we not had those experiences.

CONTENTS

ACKNOWLEDGMENTS

Many thanks to Brenda Smith Myles for her mentorship and guidance in the development of this work. She has enthusiastically supported this project and we are grateful for her ongoing support.

We appreciate the meticulous editing by Ruth Prystash. Her recommendations and insight inspired additions that enhanced the format and content of this book.

Thank you to the AAPC staff members who have worked diligently to bring this book to publication.

We are also very grateful to our families for their ongoing love and support throughout this project.

FOREWORD

"... a student with EF difficulties may find it tough to achieve in school, not because of a lack of effort or desire to do well but due to a lack of the necessary skills. Often these students are seen as unmotivated or behaviorally challenged. However, it is important to differentiate between 'won't' and 'can't.' Although it may seem as though a student could meet expectations if she wanted to, but doesn't do so because she simply won't, perhaps the reality is that she lacks the skills to do what is expected and, therefore, cannot meet the expectations without support (Wilkins & Burmeister, 2015, p. 9)."

I know it is highly unusual to quote book authors in a foreword, but Wilkins and Burmeister succinctly explain the importance of learning, highlighting the challenges that a student with executive function difficulties experiences.

What skills are most important to life success? While the list may be long, some of the most important skills include:

1. Flexibility. Things change often and quickly in life and we must be able to adapt.
2. Leveled emotionality. We need to remain calm when we should, with our emotions and behavior matching our environment.
3. Impulse control. It is important to think before acting.
4. Planning. It is important to know what to do next and next and next.
5. Problem solving. Life can be considered one big problem – from not being able to find your left shoe to not remembering where you parked your car in the parking lot. How and when you solve problems is important.

These skills fall under the rubric of executive function. And if you have these skills, your life is likely to be more successful than if you did not. Good executive function skills lead to success at home, school, work and community. They also lead to success in making friends, working with colleagues, and having a romantic relationship.

This marvelous book discusses how to teach these pivotal skills to students across the age range. In addition, the authors illustrate how teaching these specific skills in childhood and adolescence impacts adulthood.

If I were to buy one book this year, this would be it!

Brenda Smith Myles, Ph.D.
Autism Consultant

CHAPTER 1
CREATING A BLUEPRINT FOR LEARNER SUCCESS

When Joey finished high school a few years ago, it was a major event. Family members and friends attended the ceremony, and his parents were proud and relieved that their son had successfully finished high school. After the ceremony, when Joey's favorite aunt asked about his plans, everyone was excited to hear that he planned on attending the local community college in a certificate program for computer technology. His parents, knowing his love of computer gaming, felt that the certificate program would be a good fit for him and would maximize his skills and interests.

Joey connected with his local Vocational Rehabilitation office, where he was assigned a VR counselor and received financial support to attend college. He was further instructed to connect with the disability services office at the college. However, Joey didn't want other students to know that he was different, so he decided not to take advantage of disability services. Into the semester, when he missed several classes, Joey's parents began to worry about his progress. He received failing grades at mid-term, due to many missed classes and numerous missing assignments. By the end of the semester, Joey decided that he didn't like attending the community college, telling his parents that the teachers didn't care about him, other students were mean and unfair, and assignments were too difficult. Joey said he'd find a job at a gaming shop.

It has now been three years since Joey left the community college, and his main daily activity is gaming. In the first year after dropping out of college, he applied for jobs at local gaming shops. Unfortunately, there were no openings, so Joey was unable to get a job in his preferred field. His VR counselor told him that he needed to complete 25 online applications each week for entry-level positions in a variety of fields. Joey struggled to complete the applications, but interviewed at over a dozen companies without success, until he eventually was hired at a fast-food restaurant.

He disliked working at the restaurant because he said it was smelly, noisy, and chaotic. His coworkers seemed to get along with each other, but Joey struggled to make a connection with them, and when he overheard a couple of co-workers making fun of him and calling him "weird" one day, he left and never went back.

Joey was hired at a drugstore after another three months of applications and interviews. He enjoyed working there, but struggled with arriving at work on time and showing up for every shift. When Joey had been late three times in a row, he received a warning and was later written up when the *manager had to call him because it was 30 minutes past his start time. Joey had forgotten to write down his work shifts and didn't realize that his shifts would change from week to week. The final straw occurred when he told a customer to leave him alone when he was stocking shelves. The manager told Joey's VR worker that Joey's irresponsibility, odd social skills, and lack of flexibility made it impossible for him to remain in the position.*

It has now been six more months since Joey's last job. His parents are very frustrated that Joey is sitting at home playing video games day after day without any kind of plan for the future. In addition, because he didn't meet the requirements for finding a job and staying in contact with the VR counselor, Joey was dropped from the program. Joey's parents are worried that he will spend the rest of his life lonely and unmotivated, and they wonder what they can do to improve the outlook for his future.

Although Joey's story is difficult to read, it is not uncommon for young adults with autism to experience similar challenges. Often the skills that students learn in school fail to translate to skills that are necessary for success in the adult world. Furthermore, many students with autism experience difficulties in generalizing the skills they have learned in one setting to novel situations (Simpson & Myles, 2007).

If Joey had learned the skills and strategies described in the following chapters, his story would look like the scenario at the end of this chapter. In that scenario, Joey is able to use executive function strategies independently to address his challenges, allowing him to enjoy a more productive and successful life.

Despite the inherent difficulties in preparing students with autism for adult life, many young people with autism are navigating the post-school world successfully. The good news is that the skills that can support success in adulthood can be taught, and generalization of skills can be achieved. In this book, you will find strategies built upon evidence-based practices in the field of autism that can support efforts to prepare children with ASD for a successful experience once they leave K-12 education.

Who Will Benefit From This Book?

Are you an educator of students from elementary to high school age? Do you work with students on the autism spectrum or with related disabilities, in general education or special education settings? Do you have students who...

- Are disorganized, messy, and constantly running late?
- Struggle with prioritizing?
- Have a tough time transitioning between activities?
- Lack time management skills?
- Have difficulty with social situations?
- Exhibit excessive emotional reactions?
- Struggle to get started and stay focused on assignments?

- Blurt out answers and disrupt classroom teaching and learning?
- Have a hard time generalizing learned skills to new environments?
- Fail to complete and/or turn in homework?
- Avoid new activities or challenging work?
- Exhibit challenging behaviors?

Do you find yourself losing sleep thinking about what might happen in the future for these students, and wondering what you might do to help them succeed in school and in future life? If so, this book is for you!

What Are Executive Function Skills?

Many educators who work with students with autism have heard the term "executive function." In fact, executive function deficits are closely linked with students with autism. However, even though EF is often discussed in individualized education program (IEP) meetings and identified as a deficit in multidisciplinary reports, many educators are unclear about what skills are included under the heading of EF. Furthermore, there is a great deal of confusion regarding which strategies best support the development of EF skills.

In the book *FLIPP the Switch: Strengthen Executive Function Skills* (Wilkins & Burmeister, 2015), EF skills are described as a group of mental processes that aid individuals in virtually all areas. Cooper-Kahn and Dietzel (2017) define executive function as "a set of processes that all have to do with managing oneself and one's resources in order to achieve a goal." Strong EF skills are associated with increased mental flexibility and decreased emotional volatility. Individuals with good EF skills are able to organize, problem-solve, plan, and focus on and remember details.

There are many EF skills that are important, and there is no agreed-upon list of EF components. In *FLIPP the Switch*, Wilkins and Burmeister organized common EF skills using the acronym FLIPP: Flexibility, Leveled Emotionality, Impulse Control, Planning/Organizing, and Problem Solving (see Figure 1.1). For example, everyone agrees that working memory is critical, and although it is not one of the five in *FLIPP the Switch*, it is incorporated throughout those EF skills. Within *FLIPP the Switch*, strategies that can be implemented by both educators and parents to strengthen EF skills in students and children are detailed.

Mastering EF skills during school years is critical to successful adulthood. Highlighting the EF components in *FLIPP the Switch,* this book illustrates how adults who learn these skills will be able to generalize them to new environments. In *FLIPP 2.0*, strategies are more complex, and instructions for implementation reflect this level of complexity. In addition, specific instructions are included for building student independence in using the strategies, with the goal of supporting students in using strategies independently as they become more self-reliant.

What Happens When EF Skills Are Underdeveloped?

A long-term study of over 11,000 kindergarten students followed three components of EF: working memory, cognitive flexibility, and inhibitory control. Researchers found that children who exhibited EF problems in kindergarten were more likely to experience academic struggles in their school years (Barshay, 2018). These struggles occurred regardless of students' backgrounds or academic abilities.

	Flexibility	The ability to change your mind and make changes to your plans as needed
	Leveled Emotionality	The ability to emotionally self-regulate and avoid extensive mood swings
	Impulse Control	The ability to control your impulses, such as waiting to speak until called upon
	Planning/Organizing	The ability to make plans and keep track of time and materials so that work is finished on time
	Problem Solving	The ability to know when there is a problem that needs to be solved, generate solutions, select one, and evaluate the outcome

Figure 1.1. Executive function skills, from: *FLIPP the Switch: Strengthen Executive Function Skills (Wilkins, Burmeister, 2015).*

When students experience challenges in the area of EF, they may struggle in a variety of areas--at school, at home, in the community, and in the workplace (Coyne & Rood, 2011). EF deficits can lead to poor planning and prioritization, difficulty with sustaining effort and completing tasks, and challenges with socialization and adaptation to change. As Figure 1.2 illustrates,

> "... a student with EF difficulties may find it tough to achieve in school, not because of a lack of effort or desire to do well but due to a lack of the necessary skills. Often these students are seen as unmotivated or behaviorally challenged. However, it is important to differentiate between 'won't' and 'can't.' Although it may seem as though a student could meet expectations if she wanted to, but doesn't do so because she simply won't, perhaps the reality is that she lacks the skills to do what is expected and, therefore, cannot meet the expectations without support (Wilkins & Burmeister, 2015, p. 9)."

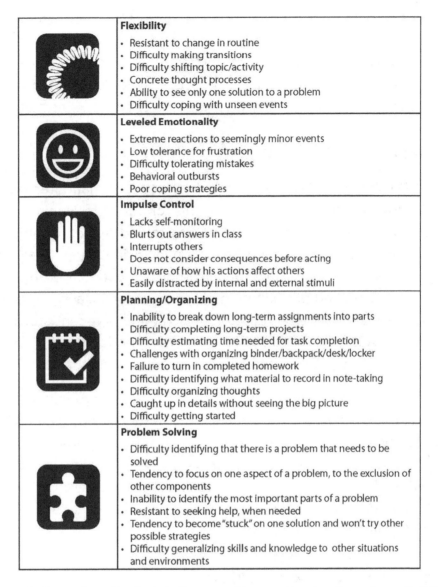

Flexibility

- Resistant to change in routine
- Difficulty making transitions
- Difficulty shifting topic/activity
- Concrete thought processes
- Ability to see only one solution to a problem
- Difficulty coping with unseen events

Leveled Emotionality

- Extreme reactions to seemingly minor events
- Low tolerance for frustration
- Difficulty tolerating mistakes
- Behavioral outbursts
- Poor coping strategies

Impulse Control

- Lacks self-monitoring
- Blurts out answers in class
- Interrupts others
- Does not consider consequences before acting
- Unaware of how his actions affect others
- Easily distracted by internal and external stimuli

Planning/Organizing

- Inability to break down long-term assignments into parts
- Difficulty completing long-term projects
- Difficulty estimating time needed for task completion
- Challenges with organizing binder/backpack/desk/locker
- Failure to turn in completed homework
- Difficulty identifying what material to record in note-taking
- Difficulty organizing thoughts
- Caught up in details without seeing the big picture
- Difficulty getting started

Problem Solving

- Difficulty identifying that there is a problem that needs to be solved
- Tendency to focus on one aspect of a problem, to the exclusion of other components
- Inability to identify the most important parts of a problem
- Resistant to seeking help, when needed
- Tendency to become "stuck" on one solution and won't try other possible strategies
- Difficulty generalizing skills and knowledge to other situations and environments

Figure 1.2. Examples of typical challenges with executive functions, from: *FLIPP the Switch: Strengthen Executive Function Skills* (Wilkins & Burmeister, 2015).

It is important to remember that individuals on the autism spectrum may exhibit both relative weaknesses and relative strengths in EF skills. As we choose strategies to use with these students, we need to make sure that we are concentrating on student strengths, while implementing strategies that will provide support for skills that are lacking. In addition, it is helpful to keep the following points in mind:

- Students with EF deficits may struggle in many areas and situations, not because they are not trying hard, but because they lack the necessary skills.
- It may be tempting to view these students as behavior problems, or unmotivated, rather than in need of instruction and environmental supports.

- We need to differentiate between "I won't" and "I can't," in order to select and implement effective strategies.
- Many students with EF deficits also demonstrate slower than normal processing speeds, which may be interpreted as stubbornness or resistance to directives. Instead, these students may need additional time to process instructions and choose the most appropriate response.

Why Do Executive Function Skills Matter?

The Individuals with Disabilities Education Act of 2004 (IDEA) mandates that schools provide transition services to prepare students with disabilities for adult life. However, research indicates that many of these students, especially those with autism and related disabilities, struggle once they leave high school. In fact, young adults with autism have difficulty with most of the outcomes their peers pursue after school, such as continuing their education, getting and keeping a job, living on their own, socializing and participating in the community, and staying healthy and safe (Roux, Shattuck, Rast, Rava, & Anderson, 2015). For example, a recent study showed that only 14% of young adults with ASD had found paid employment, and 25% of the group were not participating in any activities (Roux, Rast, Anderson, & Shattuck, 2017).

Being employed, living independently, and participating in the community are a "rite of passage" for young adults and are considered a mark of success. However, more than 85% of young adults with ASD struggle to find employment and consequently lack the financial resources to participate in other typical adult activities (Roux et al., 2015). These young adults and their families often do not know where to turn, and question why they were not better prepared in their school programs. For their part, educators work tirelessly to teach these students, and wonder how to better prepare them for life after school.

How Do We Teach Executive Function Skills?

Throughout their school years, *all* individuals with ASD will require direct instruction in skills other than academics (Myles, Aspy, Mataya, & Shaffer, 2018). Students need to be assessed for mastery of EF skills just as they would for any other subject. These skills must then be strategically and explicitly taught in order to build executive function skills that lead to greater success for these students in school and post-school life.

Explicit instruction has been defined as instruction that utilizes supports (sometimes called scaffolds) to guide students through the learning process (Archer & Hughes, 2011). Providing clear explanations regarding the purpose or rationale for learning the skill, detailed demonstrations of the steps involved in learning the skill, and assistance (including feedback) until the skill is mastered, are hallmarks of explicit instruction.

Archer and Hughes (2011) describe six ways that instruction can be scaffolded to provide support for students learning a new skill:

1. Break complex skills into manageable chunks and teach each piece to mastery.

2. Sequence skills logically.
3. Provide increasingly complex examples.
4. Model the skill and provide an example of the completed product.
5. Prompt students as they practice the new skill.
6. Use aids, such as visual prompts, to support memorization of steps used to finish tasks.

In this book, we will use scaffolding strategies to provide detailed instruction for learners at three stages of mastery. The following icons will be used throughout the book to identify level of scaffolding, based on individual student needs.

Stage 1 Learners   Stage One learners are those who are in need of the highest support. In this stage, the teacher will provide the greatest level of oversight and practice will be more controlled and specific.

Stage 2 Learners   Stage Two learners are those who are becoming more independent in their learning of the skill. At this stage, students will work in small groups to practice skills, and will have opportunities to generalize their skills with support.

Stage 3 Learners   Stage Three learners are working on generalizing their skills to new environments. At this stage, teachers are still providing support, in the form of coaching around planning and reflection, as well as data-collection and review.

How Do Evidence-Based Practices Support EF Skills?

Each of our students enters our classrooms with a unique set of characteristics and circumstances that affect their learning. No two students on the autism spectrum are alike or need the exact same types of supports and interventions. Over the past 20 years, prevalence estimates of individuals identified with ASD have reflected continuing increases in the number of students who need special educational services. Within that same period of time in the US, passage of national legislation, such as the NCLB (No Child Left Behind) Act of 2001, compelled teachers to use evidence-based practices (EBPs), which can be defined as interventions that have scientific evidence proving their effectiveness (Odom et al., 2005).

The good news is that educators now have a wide range of resources to inform and guide their efforts. Specifically, focused intervention practices that have substantial evidence for effectiveness in promoting positive outcomes for learners with ASD have been identified. Three reports that have established effective interventions for individuals with ASD include the review of the National Standards Project (NSP), completed by the National Autism Center (NAC) (National Autism Center, 2015); the National Professional Development Center (NPDC) on Autism Spectrum Disorders (ASD) (Wong et al., 2014); and the Centers for Medicare and Medicaid Services (CMMS 2010).

All three reviews applied rigorous criteria in determining which studies to include as efficacy for a given practice, providing comprehensive information about the level of scientific evidence that exists in support of the many educational treatments available for individuals with ASD. Although the findings in each review are somewhat different (e.g., the NSP defined its unit of analysis as "treatments," whereas the NPDC identified its unit as "focused intervention practices"), there is much overlap between the three reviews and many of the same practices are identified in each. Evidence-based practices, as identified by the NAC, NPDC, and CMS, are illustrated in Table 1.1.

Evidence-Based Practice	CMS		NAC		NPDC	
	Elementary	Secondary	Elementary	Secondary	Elementary	Secondary
Antecedent-Based Interventions	X	X	X	X	X	X
Behavioral Package	X		X	X	X	X
• Differential Reinforcement					X	X
• Extinction					X	X
• Reinforcement					X	X
• Discrete Trial Training					X	
• Time Delay					X	X
• Response Interruption/Redirection					X	
• Naturalistic Teaching Strategies					X	
• Picture Exchange Communication System					X	
• Pivotal Response Training®					X	
• Cognitive Behavioral Package	X		X		X	X
• Functional Behavior Assessment					X	X
• Functional Communication Training	X				X	X
• Task Analysis					X	
Exercise					X	X
Joint Attention Intervention	X		X			
Modeling	X		X		Video Modeling	Video Modeling
Multi-Component Package	X				X	
Parent-Implemented Interventions			X		X	
Peer-Implemented Interventions	X		X		X	X
Self-Management	X		X	X	X	X
Social Interventions	X			X	X	
• Social Communication Intervention	X					
• Social Skills Package	X			X	X	
• Social Skills Training	X				X	X
• Structured Play Groups	X				X	
Social Narratives/Story-Based Intervention Package	X		X		X	X
Structured Teaching	X					
• Schedules	X		X			
• Visual supports	X				X	X
Technology-Based Treatment/Technology-Aided Instruction and Intervention	X				X	X

Table 1.1. Evidence-based practices identified by the National Autism Center (NAC), National Professional Development Center (NPDC), and Centers for Medicare and Medicaid Services (CMS).
From: *Excelling with Autism: Obtaining critical mass using deliberate practice*, (Myles, Aspy, Mataya, & Shaffer, 2018).

The NAC and NPDC, as well as CMS, have taken the initial steps in helping educators learn how to improve outcomes for students with ASD by identifying which practices are evidence-based (Marder & deBettencourt, 2015). Training educators on how to select and implement these EBPS within their classrooms and other school settings is a critical component in improving current dismal post-school outcomes for many students. Training and support of teachers on how to implement evidence-based practices (EBPs) is the most efficient way for schools to provide effective educational settings for the growing number of students with ASD (Alexander, Ayres, & Smith, 2015). Unfortunately, teachers and others who support students with autism, including paraprofessionals, school psychologists, and additional related service personnel, do not always get the proper training and follow-up to become well-versed in evidence-based practices and how to implement them.

How Can This Book Help?

Most educational programs emphasize academic achievement, but business owners and college professors have made it clear that EF skills are crucial to success in the adult world (Hedley et al., 2017; Dipedeo, Storlie & Johnson, 2015). Just as academic skills must be directly and explicitly taught, EF skills need to be taught, practiced, and monitored in order for students to be able to generalize them into the real world.

This book can be a valuable personnel preparation resource for educating students with autism, helping to ensure that the content of educational programs for students with ASD is based on sound research. When best practices are implemented with fidelity, student outcomes improve (Marder & deBettencourt, 2015). This book empowers educators to use EBPs in building class-rooms designed to increase executive function skills, which not only improves student outcomes in school, but also increases the likelihood of success during transition and adult life.

FLIPP 2.0 provides a blueprint for identifying the skills that students need for future success, along with specific strategies that will support students in building strong, long-term gains in executive function skills. The remainder of the book presents this information as follows. In Chapter 2, you will learn how to design an effective educational environment that will support positive behavior and foster learning. Chapter 3 provides information on how to maximize instructional time by using effective procedures and routines. Chapter 4 focuses on how to design effective instruction for large and small groups, including the use of visual supports and structured activities and tasks to increase student engagement. Chapter 5 builds on the foundational information in Chapters 2, 3, and 4 by presenting tools that can be used to more deeply understand underlying causes of challenging behavior, leading to more effective behavioral interventions. Finally, Chapter 6 pro-vides specific information on how to reinforce the EF skills that have been mastered to prepare students for a successful transition into adult life.

Each chapter is organized as follows:

- An opening scenario consisting of real-life examples of students with challenges that you may find familiar.

- A description of the chapter topic area and the focus for each executive function skill in that chapter.
- An overview of evidence-based practices that can be implemented to increase executive function skills and support positive behavior.
- Strategies and tools to teach and support executive function skills, with specific implementation guidelines.
- Data collection tools to measure the success of strategies, with examples of completed forms, plus templates for all forms in the appendices.
- Additional scenarios that illustrate the concepts, and examples of how educators have implemented them.

Remember Joey, from the first scenario in this chapter? You may recall that Joey struggled following high school. He was unprepared for the challenges of adult life, as he had never been taught basic EF skills during his school career. Let's look at an alternate future for Joey, one in which he is reaping the benefits of a well-crafted educational program across all grades—one in which EF skills were emphasized and taught.

When Joey finished high school a few years ago, it was a major event. Family members and friends attended the ceremony, and Joey's parents were proud that he had successfully finished high school. After the ceremony, they gathered for a celebration to honor not only Joey, but also some of the staff who supported Joey during his kindergarten through high school experiences. Joey's kindergarten teacher taught him the importance of sharing classroom materials with others, and waiting appropriately to take his turn during activities. By the second grade, Joey had become impulsive and struggled to pay attention in class, but the teacher arranged the classroom in a way that allowed him to have flexible seating choices and helped him maintain focus. Joey's fourth-grade teachers partnered with his parents to support Joey in developing healthy homework habits that carried him through middle school and high school. In upper elementary grades, visual supports helped Joey learn to control his emotions. Although Joey worried that these supports might make him stand out as he got older, when he transitioned to middle school, many of his teachers were using visual supports as a class-wide strategy, and individual visual tools were available to any student who needed them, whether or not they had an IEP. Joey did not feel embarrassed about using supports, and he became independent in using several visual strategies that he kept in his binder and on his phone. In the seventh grade, an instructional assistant in his language arts class taught him to organize his paperwork in a binder, and followed through with a weekly binder check until Joey was successfully organizing his materials independently. Joey's eleventh grade intervention teacher encouraged Joey to set meaningful goals, and taught him how to break long term school projects down into manageable pieces, in order to complete the work on time. Each of these educators had helped Joey acquire the EF skills that enabled him to succeed in high school.

Joey's family members were excited to learn that he planned on attending the local community college in a certificate program for computer technology. Knowing his love of anything related to computers, Joey's parents felt that the certificate program would be a good fit for him and would maximize his skills and interests.

Following graduation, Joey connected with his local Vocational Rehabilitation (VR) office, where he was assigned a VR counselor and received financial support to attend college. His VR counselor also instructed him to connect with the disability services office at the college. Joey understood that even though it had required hard work on his part, much of his school success so far was due to the specialized services he had received because of his disability. Therefore, he took advantage of the disability services offered at the college, and found that he not only received support to help him in his coursework, but also had access to information for gaining experience in his chosen field of study through partnerships with local businesses.

Joey found a posting for an intern position in the Information Technology and Support Services Department in his hometown. Although this would be an unpaid position, Joey was interested in his city's government, and he thought he would enjoy learning more about this department. Joey applied and was accepted for the position, and when he had completed his intern hours, the department was so pleased with Joey's work that they created a part-time job for him. Once he received his college degree, Joey was hired in a full-time position by the city as an IT specialist in media services. After completing one year in this position, Joey was selected as the city employee of the year. At the celebration held to present this award, city staff acknowledged the attributes that Joey brings to his work: the ability to prioritize, plan and organize, problem solve, manage time and meet deadlines, work well with others and consider multiple perspectives, and demonstrate flexibility – in other words, Joey does what needs to be done to successfully accomplish any task.

Joey looks forward to going to work every day. Joey's family and friends are thrilled with his new career, and excited for the possibilities ahead of him. Everyone encounters new challenges in work and in life, and so will Joey, but he knows that he now has the tools to deal with those challenges as he moves forward.

CHAPTER 2
DESIGNING THE ENVIRONMENT TO SUPPORT LEARNING

*M*r. Gallegos is experiencing a combination of excitement and a slight sense of trepidation as he prepares for his class this year. This is his first year of teaching elementary students, and he has agreed to take on a co-teaching role with an experienced special educator and seven students with IEPs. In addition, there are five students who are English language learners in his room.

Mr. Gallegos has decided the best way to engage his class is to have a Jumanji theme for the year. He spent the week before the beginning of school making his class into a jungle. He covered the windows with green paper and made dozens of brightly colored flowers, which he attached to the walls. In the reading corner, he made a papier maché coconut palm tree, complete with swaying branches and hanging coconuts. He also hung tropical birds and monkeys from the ceiling. In fact, Mr. Gallegos was so busy setting up his classroom that he missed the meeting with his co-teacher. But he's sure it will be fine; after all, how hard can it be? He has decided it will be helpful for his students to work in groups, so Mr. Gallegos changed from rows to round tables that are spread around the room. He has decided to allow the students to choose their own groups on the first day.

On the morning of the first day of school, Mr. Gallegos excitedly greets his students as they come in the door. He is pleased to hear shrieks of delight at seeing the jungle. Unfortunately, some of the children do not seem to be pleased, which he does not understand. In fact, one student pulls his shirt over his head and sits in the corner crying and rocking back and forth. Mr. Gallegos thinks this student should not be in his class and plans to bring this up with his co-teacher as soon as possible. Admittedly, it did get a little chaotic when the students did not know where to sit, and when one of them, Jordan, tried to climb the coconut tree. It didn't help that his co-teacher, Ms. Khouri, kept asking him what the lesson plan was for the day, where the students should sit, and how she could support him. In addition, she clearly did not seem to be excited about the Jumanji theme.

After lunch, Ms. Khouri gathers the students with IEPs and pulls them into a corner for a reading activity. However, finding it is too noisy for them to concentrate, she ends up taking the group into the hallway to complete their activity.

Mr. Gallegos is surprised by his students' behavior. He can't understand why they are so noisy and out of control all day. He thought teaching kids in a jungle theme environment would be invigorating, but instead it was exhausting. He is also sad because his beautiful room is looking a little worse for wear by the end of the day.

Luckily, following the hectic first day of class, he has an opportunity to talk with his co-teacher, who has some suggestions regarding how to structure the environment to support positive behavior. Together they work to make the classroom less busy, and more conducive for learning. They also spend time thinking about the kind of learning activities they will be utilizing, and planning the space strategically to accommodate those learning activities. Despite his initial disappointment and confusion, looking at the classroom at the beginning of the second day of school, Mr. Gallegos reflects on how lucky he is to be able to plan with another teacher with a wealth of knowledge and experience. He is now looking forward to the collaboration with Ms. Khouri for the remainder of the year.

As adults, we all have preferences about our living spaces. We like to have our kitchen laid out in a way that makes it easy for us to prepare meals. We don't want our living rooms too cold or too hot. We don't like seeing clutter in our bedrooms. The classroom environment is just as important, and can prove either distracting or calming. This chapter will discuss strategies to help students learn to tolerate and control their own environments. It will highlight the importance of a well-designed environment in building executive function skills, increasing learning, and supporting students in becoming more independent. You will learn five strategies that can be used to maximize the learning environment. For each of these strategies, you will learn steps to gradually give responsibility to the student, which will allow them to use the strategies independently. These strategies are not only necessary for school success, but also essential to being a successful adult at work, at home, and in the community. Thus, this chapter will also highlight the direct impact the five strategies have on everyday adult life. Blank copies of all of the tools in this chapter are also provided in Appendix A.

Link to Executive Function

Well-designed classrooms play a crucial role in keeping *all* students engaged in appropriate behaviors conducive to learning and success. This is especially important for students with EF deficits, who often have difficulty navigating unpredictable and overstimulating environments within the school. Well-structured, predictable classrooms help students understand where to sit, stand, line up, go next, where to put things, what to attend to, and which activities and choices are available. This can decrease student anxiety, increase positive behavior, provide opportunities for greater independence, and lead to an improvement in academic skills. Table 2.1 describes how a structured environment can support key EF skills, and how these skills impact adult life.

Link to Executive Function			
Areas of Executive Function	A well-structured environment provides support by:	Adults who have learned these skills will be able to:	Real-world examples of effective EF skills:
Developing flexibility	Giving students a clear and understandable design that provides a predictable and orderly environment, while also allowing for some flexibility for different learning tasks.	Adapt to changes in typical environments, including home, work, and the community, and adjust to new environments as needed.	Evaluates the workspace and makes minor changes to improve work function. Moves from one spot to another as needed, even if the preference is to stay in a certain area.
Leveling emotions	Assisting students in managing anxiety that may be exacerbated by a chaotic, cluttered, and overly stimulating environment.	Use self-regulation strategies to manage anxiety in chaotic, overly stimulating, or unpredictable environments.	Takes a break for two to three minutes (e.g., walk for three minutes; use a calming app for two minutes) to maintain appropriate level of work or social interaction.
Increasing impulse control	Arranging a space that is predictable, safe, and orderly, and providing instruction in specific strategies that can decrease impulsivity.	Recognize when the environment or part of it may result in impulsivity, and use strategies to increase a sense of safety, predictability, and order.	Finds a quiet area and uses calming strategies (e.g., headphones, pocket fidget, deep breathing).
Planning and organizing	Offering students a clear, well-planned, and organized environment that provides modifications designed to increase organizational skills.	Identify environmental elements that lead to personal success and implement modifications that result in high productivity.	Organizes work area to face away from distractions. Uses visual organizers and lists to separate and organize work projects.
Problem solving	Helping students to recognize supportive elements in the environment and identify problems when they occur.	Understand when a problem occurs in the environment, generate possible solutions, choose one, and evaluate the outcome.	Recognizes a problem situation or area, uses a process to determine possible solutions, then chooses and tries a solution and decides if it works.

Table 2.1. Link between EF skills and the environment.

Structuring the Environment and Evidence-Based Practices

A well-structured classroom works as an antecedent-based intervention, in that a properly designed instructional environment can increase learning and reduce problem behaviors through providing structure, predictability, and safety. In many cases, problem behaviors occur because there is a mismatch between the skills and strengths of the students and the environment (Kern & Clemens, 2007). In a well-designed classroom, students understand expectations and feel safe and comfort-

EBPs in this Chapter

- Antecedent-Based Intervention
- Visual Supports
- Self-Management
- Social Narratives

able. Such an environment can support students in building self-management skills through the expeditious use of well-designed visual supports (Wong et al., 2014).

Structuring the Classroom Environment

Physical characteristics of a classroom environment include such things as the amount of light in the room, the temperature and air quality, the amount of color and complexity, along with flexibility and the sense of ownership students feel in the space – all characteristics that have been shown to have an impact on academic growth in reading, writing, and mathematics (Barrett, Zhang, Davies, & Barrett, 2015). Although some characteristics of the classroom environment are beyond a teacher's direct control – the number of windows, amount of space, structural design, air quality – several other features can be modified and adjusted by the teacher to make the learning environment a more welcoming space (see Table 2.2).

Physical Characteristics of the Classroom Environment		
Component	**Description**	**What can the teacher do?**
Personal Connection	The level of individualization within the design of the classroom: • How are students connected to the space? • How can they feel a sense of ownership of the classroom? • How does the classroom strengthen the relationship between students and the teacher? • How does the classroom help students to interact with each other?	Think about how students can be a part of decorating and designing the space. • How can student work be used to decorate the room? • What is distinctive about the space? What can make it different from other classrooms in the building? • How can the classroom help students think of themselves as a cohesive group?

Adaptability	The level of adaptability in the organization and design of the room: • How easy is it to change the arrangement to allow for a variety of learning activities? • How easily can the classroom accommodate students who may need lower levels of noise, light, and movement?	Think about the different learning activities that will occur in the room. • Will the current design accommodate all of them? • If not, is it possible to rearrange the classroom to meet the learning demands?
Color and Contrast	The balance of color in the room: • The room should be neither too colorful, nor too monochromatic. • Bright colors should be used judiciously to prevent overstimulation. • Blue coloring has been found to be less distracting and more calming (Johnson & Ruiter, 2013).	Evaluate the color palette in the classroom. • Is it monochromatic, or bright and bold? Include the furniture and other features in your evaluation. • How can you use color to either brighten or calm down the space? • How can you use color to create a warm and welcoming space that is neither overstimulating nor boring?
Visual Stimulation	The amount of visual stimulation in the room. • The room should not be overly decorated to prevent creating a sense of chaos and a high level of visual distraction. • On the other hand, the space needs to be visually interesting and capable of stimulating students' attention. Items such as soft chairs, pillows, rugs, and plants can provide visual stimulation and add comfort and warmth to the classroom (Rutter, Maughan, Mortimore, & Ouston, 1979).	Keep in mind that too much visual distraction can be as detrimental as too little. • How might wall space be used to create visual interest? Typically, less than 50%-80% of the wall space should be covered, depending upon the underlying design of the room. • How will you organize the visuals in the room? • Will they be changed throughout the school year? If so, how often? Will there be spaces in the room with less visual stimulation for those students who need a more calming visual environment?

Lighting	The amount and quality of the light in the room: • Is there a sufficient amount of natural light, and how will the natural light be supplemented with electric lights? • Natural light is preferable; however, electric lights are often necessary to provide additional light. • The classroom should be bright enough for students to see easily, but not so bright as to cause problems with glare.	Take a look at the amount of light available in the classroom without the fluorescent lights on. • Is enough light coming through the windows alone? Be mindful of covering the windows and reducing the amount of natural light that can enter the space. Keep in mind that the noise from fluorescent lights can disturb some students. • With this in mind, can the amount of light in the room be supplemented with lamps that feature softer, more natural light than what is offered through fluorescent lighting?
Air Quality	The amount of fresh air circulating in the room: • How is the room ventilated in order to provide fresh air?	Is the air in the room circulated via the air conditioning/heating system, or will the windows be used to incorporate fresh air into the space? • Consider using a CO_2 monitor in the room to determine whether or not the air is circulating sufficiently.
Temperature	The temperature level in the room: • Is the room a comfortable temperature, i.e., neither too cool nor too warm?	Pay attention to the orientation of the classroom and the amount of sunlight that may come through the windows, affecting the temperature of the space. • If the sun does cause the room to get too warm, use the blinds or curtains to limit the amount of direct sunlight that enters the classroom. • Consider using a thermometer to gauge the temperature in the classroom and aim for a neutral temperature – neither too warm nor too cool.

Use of Space and Organization	The physical set-up of the classroom: • How are desks, tables, chairs, and other furniture arranged in the space? • There should be enough space for students to move around easily and safely, and the teacher(s) should be able to easily monitor all areas of the classroom. • There is some indication that having students seated in rows leads to increases in academic performance (Kern & Clemens, 2007); however, many teachers feel that desks that are grouped, or having students grouped at tables, is beneficial for building a sense of community and encouraging cooperative learning (Bucholz & Sheffler, 2009).	Think about how best to design the classroom space to encourage learning. • Elementary classrooms may incorporate more grouping strategies, whereas secondary classrooms may have students seated in rows or in groups. • Consider principles of universal design, whereby spaces are designed from the outset to ensure that all materials, equipment, and activities are accessible to and usable by all students (Bucholz & Sheffler, 2009). • How can the classroom be organized to meet the needs of all students, ensuring safety and accessibility for everyone?

Table 2.2. Physical characteristics of the classroom environment. *Adapted from Barrett et al., 2015.*

Designing the Environment to Support All Learners

Though no particular arrangement of the physical environment is appropriate for all classrooms, the best setup is one that combines the unique educator and learner characteristics with a structured classroom environment. Placement of furniture and other materials helps to provide clear physical and visual boundaries in school environments by segmenting and establishing the context of that environment, and by enabling students to predict events and activities, anticipate change, understand expectations, and make sense of their environment and the behaviors that are expected within that environment (Simonsen, Fairbanks, Briesch, Myers, & Sugai, 2008).

Key strategies in designing the physical environment include structuring the classroom to facilitate typical instructional activities, positioning furniture to allow for efficient staff and student movement, ensuring the instructional materials are neat, organized, and ready for use, and displaying materials that reinforce essential content and learning strategies (Simonsen et al., 2015).

To get started, consider a classroom design that facilitates typical instructional activities with areas that are age-appropriate, address IEP goals, and incorporate standards-based academic goals, along with functional and life skills activities, if indicated. Next, add zones, or areas designated for particular activities. Students and staff may find it helpful to have labels or signs posted in some zones as a visual reminder of the activities and behavioral expectations for that area.

The *Classroom Zones Chart* (see Table 2.3) describes areas or zones that can be modified or adjusted depending on the grade or developmental level of the students in the classroom or the amount of support needed, from mild to significant. However, it is important to recognize that not all zones are essential to all classrooms. For example, students with significant support needs may benefit from transition, daily living, and movement or sensory zones, while others may not.

Classroom Zones Chart
Class Time or Whole Class
Arrangement of student desks, tables, or other classroom furniture that facilitates whole-class, teacher-led instruction where information or material is presented to all students together.
Group Zone
Teaching tables where an adult works with a small (two to three) or large (four or more) group of students. Group table work may be used for academics, social, fine motor, art and domestic skills.
Learning Centers
Areas where students engage in self-directed activities, typically involving interesting experiences to enhance learning.
One-to-One Center
Table or desk where staff works one-to-one with a particular student on direct teaching of new skills, including standards-based IEP goals.
Work Alone or Independent Work Zone
An area for independent work that is based on mastery of skills previously taught; this can include student desks with study carrels or clearly defined workstations where students work independently.
Circle or Class Meeting
An area for calendar, opening group activity, presentations, and social skills.
Play Zone or Break Area
An area where students may have the opportunity to select activities of their choice, such as preferred toys, music, magazines, games, and electronics.
Book Zone or Library Area
An area where students work alone or in small groups, with books to support academics, as well as preferred books.
Cool-Down Area or Home Base
A designated area where students can go to self-regulate during times of stress.
Movement Area or Sensory Zone
An area furnished with sensory manipulatives and movement equipment.
Snack Area or Nutrition Zone
An area that can be used to work on dining skills, such as learning to eat new foods.
Transition Center
A designated area with student schedules, and a place for taking a break, to support students whose difficult transitions between activities and poor waiting skills are negatively impacting their learning (Golden, 2012).

Daily Living Center
An area for simple food preparation, basic laundry, and classroom chores.
Vocational Skills Center
An area equipped with desks, workbenches, or tables for vocational work systems.

Table 2.3. Classroom zones or areas.

Special Education Classroom Diagram

This is an example of an elementary special education classroom (see Figure 2.1). The zones or areas for this class include:

1. Whole group or circle for new learning using the interactive white board
2. Small-group instruction for new learning and practice activities
3. One-to-one instruction for new learning
4. Work alone for independent work tasks
5. Transition Center for student schedules and a rug for taking a break to help with transitioning from place to place and activity to activity
6. Sensory/movement area for self-regulation activities
7. Tablet and listening center for practice and self-regulation activities
8. Reading/book center for read-aloud activities and independent reading
9. Labels for each area
10. Signs for classroom rules and current academic standards posted near the white board
11. Signs for classroom and behavioral routines posted throughout the classroom

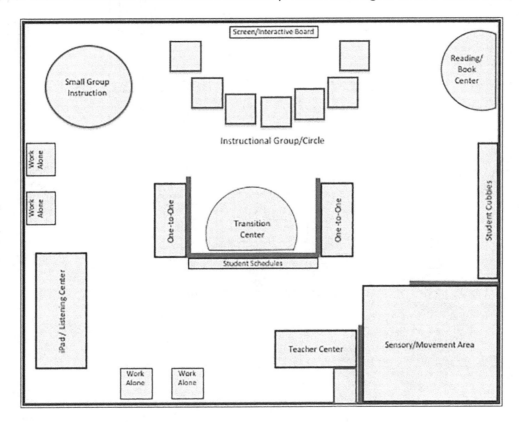

Figure 2.1. Elementary special education classroom.

Elementary Classroom Diagram

This is an example of an elementary general education classroom that also supports inclusion (see Figure 2.2). The zones or areas included in this class include:

1. Whole group/student groups for new learning using the interactive white board
2. Small-group instruction for new learning and practice activities
3. One-to-one instruction for individualized learning and behavior support
4. Tablet center for practice and self-regulation activities
5. Reading/book center for read-aloud activities and independent reading
6. Math and science centers for small-group practice activities
7. Labels for most areas
8. Signs for classroom rules and current academic standards posted near the white board
9. Signs for classroom and behavioral routines posted throughout the classroom

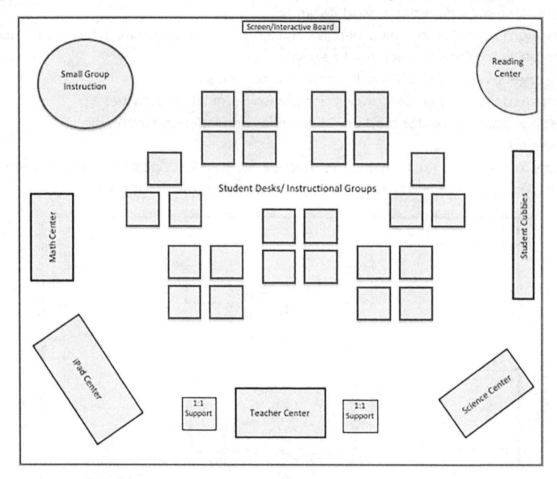

Figure 2.2. Elementary classroom.

Secondary Classroom Diagram

This is an example of a secondary general education classroom that also supports inclusion (see Figure 2.3). The zones or areas included in this class include:

1. Whole group (student desks) for new learning using the interactive white board
2. Focused small-group instruction for new learning and practice activities
3. Teacher center also used for individualized student support
4. Technology center for independent practice and research activities.
5. Signs for current academic standards, classroom rules and procedures, and behavioral routines posted in strategic places throughout the classroom, which may include: Getting Started, Tech Center Rules, Group Learning Etiquette, Cell Phone Rules, Getting Help, End-of-Class Reminders, and Homework Assignments

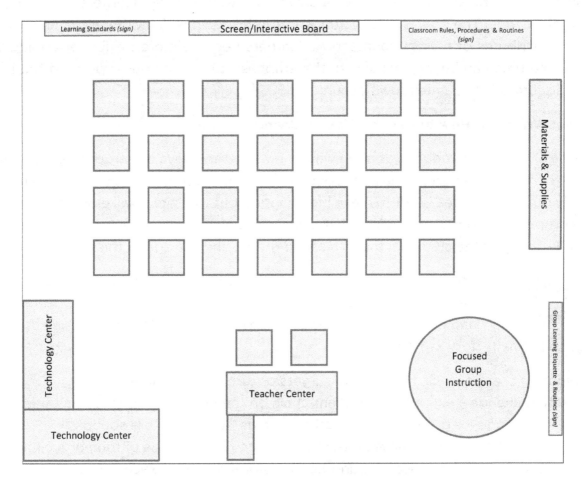

Figure 2.3. Secondary classroom.

Flexibility: *Making Changes Game*

Coping with changes in the environment may be difficult for many individuals with ASD. Dealing with new situations can be impacted by inflexibility and poor problem-solving skills (Minshew & Williams, 2008). This lack of flexibility is an indication that the student needs practice with remaining calm in a new environment or where changes have been made to a familiar environment. Providing practice in coping with new situations can be an excellent way to teach flexibility and provide positive practice in self-management skills.

 Why Is This Important?

The function of the *Making Changes Game* incorporates planned changes to the environment, a visual timer, and a reminder card to allow students to practice appropriate ways of dealing with environmental changes. It also provides a structured way to assist learners in moving outside their comfort zone. The goal is to structure short intervals in which different changes are made to certain attributes of the environment. As learners become more flexible at coping with the changes, the time can be increased, with the emphasis placed on never pushing the learner so far into discomfort that a meltdown occurs.

Teachers: When and How to Use the *Making Changes Game*

The game should be introduced as a fun way to try different ways of introducing changes within the classroom. Prior to starting the game, decide what kind of small changes could be made easily and fairly quickly. The idea is not to make big changes, but to make small environmental changes for a short period of time. In deciding what kinds of changes to make, take into consideration the level of flexibility of the students, the size of the group, and the age of the students.

Stage 1 Learners For Stage One learners, use a large reminder card to signal the start of the game (see Figure 2.4). Have students get out their *Individual Reminder Cards* and place them on their desk (see Figure 2.5). Use a die to select the type of change to be made, for example:

1. Lighting change – e.g., turn off some lights or turn on more lights.
2. Seating change – e.g., sit in a different chair, on the floor, or on chairs at a table.
3. Sound change – e.g., play music or other sounds, such as nature sounds.
4. Furniture change – e.g., move student desks into pairs, groups of four, or a circle.
5. Location change – e.g., work at another table or a different place in the room.
6. Teacher choice – e.g., any of the above or any other small environmental change.

Set the timer for one to ten minutes. Start with a very short amount of time and work up to more time as students become accustomed to dealing with changes.

Stage 2 Learners For Stage Two learners, prompt students to play the game. Have individual students roll the die to select the change and choose the amount of time. After the game is finished, have students talk about how they felt during the game.

Stage 3 Learners For Stage Three learners, students may choose new environments within the school. For students who are younger or need more oversight, have the student choose a familiar area (e.g., lunch room, library, gym) to pair with an unfamiliar activity. See *Directions for Students* below and the example *Making Changes Student Question Card* (see Figure 2.6).

Class Making Changes Game

1. Be ready for your teacher to announce that it is time to play the game.
2. One student will roll the die to show the change to be made.
3. The teacher will set the timer.
4. Students, do your best to remain calm until the timer stops.

Figure 2.4. Large whole-class reminder card for making changes game.

Individual Reminder Card:
Making Changes Game

1. I will listen for my teacher to tell me it is time to play "Making Changes."
2. My teacher will pick one student to roll the die to see what change will be made.
3. My teacher will set the timer.
4. I will do my best to stay calm and work hard until the time ends.

Figure 2.5. Individual student reminder card for making changes game.

Directions for Students

When and How You Can Use the *Making Changes Question Card*

Coping with changes can be stressful, but it is an important life skill. Learning to handle changes in the environment will take practice. Being able to practice while you have some control over the situation can make it easier to deal with changes. You can play this game with other students in the classroom, or if your teacher says it's OK, you can go to a different place on campus. Follow these directions to play the *Making Changes Game:*

- Pick a time to play the game for about five to fifteen minutes and choose a new place from a list of places on campus.
- Use the *Making Changes Question Card* (see Figure 2.6, Appendix A) to answer questions about your experience.
- As you get more comfortable with trying new places, try to spend more time in each new environment.

Making Changes Student Question Card			
Student: _____Joey_____	New Place: _____Assembly/Gym_____		
1. Where is it located?	☒ indoors	☐ outdoors	
2. What I saw:	☐ no people	☐ 1-2 people	☒ 10+ people
3. What I heard:	☒ loud noises	☐ background noise	☐ quiet
4. What I felt:	☒ anxious & stressed	☐ calm & happy	
5. How long did I stay?	☐ 5 minutes	☒ 10 minutes	☐ 30+ minutes
6. Was I comfortable?	☐ Yes	☒ No	
7. Will I go to this place again?	☒ Yes	☐ No	

Figure 2.6. Making changes student question card–example.

Data Collection

Collect data on how long individual Stage 3 learners are able to play the *Making Changes Game* and whether or not the game was initiated by the teacher or the student using the *Making Changes Game: Teacher Data Collection Chart* (see Figure 2.7, Appendix A). In the examples (see Figures 2.6 and 2.7) Joey tried two new environments, increased his time from the first to the second new environment, and completed the *Making Changes Student (MC) Question Card* for both experiences.

Making Changes Game: Teacher Data Collection Chart				
Student Name: _____Joey_____				
Date:	Type of environmental change/name of place:	Length of Time in New Environment *(minutes)*:	Initiated by: S = Student T = Teacher	*MC* Question Card Completed?
9/15	Assembly/Gym	☐ 5 ☒ 10 ☐ 30+	☒ S ☐ T	☒ yes ☐ no
9/20	Library	☐ 5 ☐ 10 ☒ 30+	☐ S ☒ T	☒ yes ☐ no
		☐ 5 ☐ 10 ☐ 30+	☐ S ☐ T	☐ yes ☐ no
		☐ 5 ☐ 10 ☐ 30+	☐ S ☐ T	☐ yes ☐ no

Figure 2.7. Making changes game data collection chart–example.

Leveled Emotionality: Strategies for Using Social Narratives

Social narratives are a type of narrative written to teach socially appropriate behaviors and responses. As an evidence-based practice that is individualized to student needs (Wong et al., 2014), they are useful for students aged preschool through adult, supporting students with a variety of learning styles in a process that can lead to more successful school experiences. They are effective tools to use with students who demonstrate behavioral outbursts, poor coping strategies, difficulty making transitions, as well as other excessive emotional reactions associated with leveled emotionality. Social narratives can be developed in various layouts that accurately describe social and/or emotional situations and provide a student with information about when something may occur, what might occur, and/or what to expect, as well as what an individual can do in a given situation (Buron & Myles, 2014). Serving as a visual cue to share accurate information, the narratives can be written by educational professionals, as well as parents, and are personalized, considering the student's age, attention span, and level of cognition.

Social narratives are developed from the perspective of the student, identifying a particular situation, providing information to assist the student in understanding the appropriate behavioral response, and identifying personal strategies to apply the information. There are a variety of media formats for presenting a social narrative. Options include a short narrative or script presented in any of the following formats:

- Typed or handwritten on paper (see Figures 2.8 and 2.10)
- Slide show such as PowerPoint
- Book created on a program such as Shutterfly
- Screen version on a tablet or a smartphone

Cartooning (see Figure 2.9), where simple drawings are used to illustrate a situation and the thoughts of others during the situation (Aspy & Grossman, 2007), can also be used in developing a social narrative. *Power Cards* are another strategy that addresses a behavior of concern by incorporating a student's highly focused interest, hero, or role model. The card contains a scenario that describes the character's problem-solving process for the behavior of concern, and a social narrative that summarizes how a student can use the same strategy to solve a similar problem (Gagnon & Myles, 2016).

 Why Is This Important?

Deficits in social awareness make appropriate interactions in social situations challenging. The function of a social narrative is to provide an individual with information regarding a social situation for which he may lack an understanding and provide a sequence or process of how to respond appropriately. Social narratives assist students in adjusting to changes in routine and adapting their behaviors based on the relevant cues of a situation, leading to increased pro-social behaviors.

Teacher Directions: When and How to Use a Social Narrative

The social narrative strategy can be used across environments including school, home, vocational, and community settings where there is a need for a social behavior to change. Social narratives can be an effective tool for students who have difficulty in school environments that they perceive as unpredictable or overstimulating, and can be individualized for use with students in all three learner stages.

| Stage 1 Learners | For Stage One learners, develop and teach the use of the social narrative by reading the narrative to or with the student and modeling the related behaviors. Have the student go through the behaviors and reinforce, or model and prompt until the student can demonstrate the behaviors. |

| Stage 2 Learners | For Stage Two learners, involve the student in developing the social narrative. Be ready to guide/remind the student to use the social narrative when you see he is being challenged by environmental problems in the classroom, on campus, or in other environments. |

| Stage 3 Learners | For Stage Three learners, as the student becomes proficient at the process, gradually release responsibility so that the use of a social narrative shifts from teacher-directed to student-directed (see *Directions for Students* below). |

| All Learners | For learners in all stages, have the narrative available for referencing as needed. Adults, as well as peers, can be involved in implementing the strategy. |

Directions for Students

When and How You Can Use a Social Narrative

- You can use social narratives independently as a strategy to manage stress and frustration.
- Social narratives can be kept in your reminder binder, in a folder in your backpack, on an electronic device, or in a place at school where you can easily reach them.
- When you are having difficulty managing your emotions at school, you can choose a social narrative that fits the situation and read it.

How to Make a Social Narrative

The content of the social narrative may be developed by a parent or education professional, and can also be created in conjunction with the student. Consider age-appropriateness, as well as developmentally appropriate language and visual supports. A narrative written for a young child may have just a few sentences; for an older individual, a narrative may be longer, as his/her attention dictates. Illustrations such as photographs, hand-drawn pictures, and computer-generated icons may be included to enhance the understanding of the expected behaviors (Wragge, 2011). The following steps outline the process for developing a social narrative at school:

- Identify a situation regarding the school environment for intervention.
- Define the expected behavior or skill.
- Determine the format for the narrative.
- Develop the narrative.

The narrative should include a statement about the problem the student is experiencing, statements about possible strategies that might help, and a statement about possible positive outcomes. These statements typically use words or phrases such as, "I will try," or "I can." It is important not to write the narrative with absolutes, as some students may experience different degrees of success, and it is important that the student never feel discouraged, only empowered to attempt to remedy the situation.

Going to the Science Center in My Classroom

 My classroom has several zones.

 My favorite zone is the science center. I can use a magnifying glass to observe minerals in rocks, or use the microscope to observe the cells in a plant.

 I can go to the science center **after** I finish my work in the independent work zone.

 It is important to stay in the independent work zone until my work is finished.

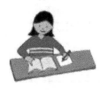 I will try to finish my work in the independent work zone so that I can go to the science center.

Figure 2.8. Social narrative in a story format with illustrations. Images ©LessonPix Inc. Used with permission.

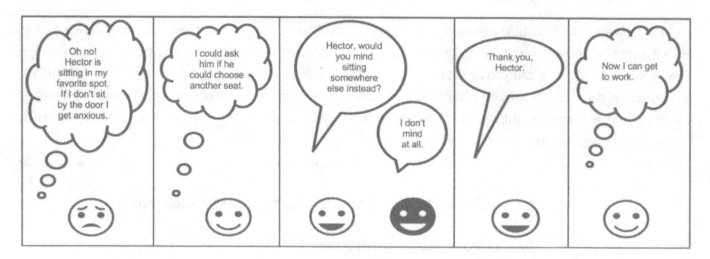

Figure 2.9. Social narrative using cartooning.

REGULATING MY BEHAVIOR IN A NOISY CLASSROOM

SOMETIMES, THE NOISE LEVEL IN MY CLASSROOM MAKES IT HARD FOR ME TO FOCUS, MAKING ME FEEL UPSET.

WHEN THAT HAPPENS:

⇨ I STOP AND TAKE A DEEP BREATH.

⇨ I TELL MYSELF, "I CAN BE FLEXIBLE! I CAN USE MY STRATEGIES."

⇨ I CAN TAKE AN ITEM FROM MY FIDGET BOX AND USE IT.

⇨ I CAN BREATHE AND COUNT TO TEN.

IF I STILL CAN'T FOCUS, I CAN ASK MY TEACHER IF I CAN WORK IN THE COMMON ROOM THAT SEPARATES THE CLASSROOMS IN MY POD.

USING THESE STRATEGIES CAN HELP ME TO REMAIN CALM AND FINISH MY WORK WHEN NOISE BOTHERS ME.

Figure 2.10. Social narrative in a story format.

Data Collection

Collect data to measure the effectiveness of the social narrative strategy with the *Using Social Narratives Data Collection Chart* (see Figure 2.11, Appendix A). Depending on the behavior that is being targeted, use the data to determine whether the strategy is effectively increasing desired behavior and/or decreasing interfering behavior. In this example, Kyle's success increased as he used the social narrative for transitioning from activity to activity (see Figure 2.11).

Using Social Narratives Data Collection Chart				
Student Name: Kyle				
Target Behavior: Transition without protest from preferred to nonpreferred activity				
Date:	**Situation:**	**Used Narrative?** Y / N	**Target Behavior Exhibited?** Y / N	**Comments:**
9/16	Going from computer to math	☑ yes ☐ no	☑ yes ☐ no	used fidget
9/18	Recess to writing group	☐ yes ☑ no	☐ yes ☑ no	Protested – refused to use strategy
9/19	Recess to writing group	☑ yes ☐ no	☑ yes ☐ no	used deep breathing strategy & count to 10
		☐ yes ☐ no	☐ yes ☐ no	
		☐ yes ☐ no	☐ yes ☐ no	

Figure 2.11. Social narrative data collection chart–example.

Impulse Control: *SOS Strategy*

Sixth-grade student Jamal was in the school conference room attending a meeting for the Science Club. He was excited about this meeting because they were going to start a new project making windmills and would be giving a kit of materials out to members of the club. As he was waiting for the other students to arrive, he began to feel jumpy and got out of his seat to wander around the room. His friend asked what was wrong, and Jamal said the room was bothering him. After 15 minutes in the room, Jamal was pacing and making noises. When Jamal flipped one of the windmill kits off of the table, his friend went to get help from the teacher. She talked to Jamal and together they figured out that the air conditioning was making a low whining sound that was causing him to feel anxious and uneasy.

Impulse control is a critical skill for many students with autism that can tip the balance between success and failure at school in both academic and social situations. Environmental factors that negatively affect a student's sensory system (sounds, smells, visual stimuli, etc.) can cause a loss of impulse control. For Jamal, understanding how to gain and maintain his impulse control will allow him to successfully function in different environments, including the Science Club.

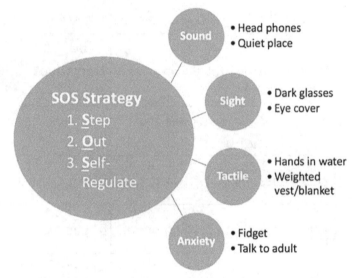

Figure 2.12. SOS strategy.

Using the *SOS Strategy* (**S**tep **O**ut & **S**elf-regulate) will give students like Jamal, who become dysregulated by environmental factors, a way to identify and handle those situations before they lose control. The *SOS Strategy* prompts the student to identify when he begins to feel anxious and then to leave the situation, going to a safe place where he can self-regulate (see Figure 2.12).

 Why Is This Important?

The function of SOS is to assist the student in controlling his behavior when environmental factors cause dysregulation and loss of impulse control. SOS gives the student a set of steps to identify the environmental problem, leave the situation for a safe place, and proactively use a tool to regain self-regulation. The goal is for the student to be an active participant in maintaining his self-regulation in order to function successfully in challenging environments.

Teacher Directions: When and How to Use SOS

Help the student identify when the environment is causing dysregulation. This should start as a structured lesson using familiar examples students can understand or have experienced. Move on to using actual problems as they occur in classroom or campus environments. Once students are familiar with SOS, use it as a proactive strategy. Remind students how to use the steps to go to a safe place and use their "tools." Provide an SOS card (see Figure 2.13) that is appropriate to the student's needs and abilities, such as:

- Make SOS into an index card or business card (as a portable and discreet visual reminder of the steps).
- Store the SOS card steps on an electronic device.

SOS Strategy

- **Step**
- **Out**
- **Self-Regulate**

Figure 2.13. SOS card.

Stage 1 Learners

For Stage One learners, introduce the SOS steps to the student using the SOS graphic. Be sure the student understands the term, "self-regulation." Show him the SOS card and go over each prompt. Use simulated situations and role-play to directly teach, reinforce, practice, and reteach each step of the process until the student can use the SOS card with minimal support. For most students, the most difficult part of the process will be identifying when they are becoming dysregulated because of an environmental factor.

Stage 2 Learners

For Stage Two learners, create or find environmental challenges in the classroom or on campus. Model using the steps to recognize and leave the situation, go to a safe place and use a tool to gain self-regulation, using a "think-aloud" process. Next, have students work in pairs to discuss how they would use the SOS card in different situations. Be ready to guide/remind the students to use the SOS process when you see they are being challenged by environmental problems in the classroom, on campus, or in other environments.

Stage 3 Learners

For Stage Three learners, as the student becomes proficient at using SOS, she will independently use the steps as described in the *Directions for Students* below.

All Learners

For learners in all stages, encourage students to recall environmental problems in other settings and what actions have been effective in those settings in order to promote generalization.

Directions for Students

When and How to Use SOS

You can use the SOS process independently to handle problems at school. Choose a place to keep the SOS card, such as:

- in your reminder binder or a folder in your backpack,
- on your electronic device,
- in a spot in your class or another place with easy access.

When you feel stressed or anxious because of something in your classroom, use the *SOS Strategy* by leaving the situation, going to a safe place, and using your tools to self-regulate. After you use the strategy, it's a good idea to debrief with your teacher so you both are aware of how you handled the problem.

 Data Collection

Use the *SOS Strategy Data Collection* tool to record how students use the *SOS Strategy* (see Figure 2.14, Appendix A). As shown in the class example below, it is important to collect data on what support students need to manage environmental challenges (see Figure 2.14).

			Prompts Needed:
Date	Student Name	Describe Environmental Challenge: Location/Sensory Impact	I = Indirect D = Direct N = None
10/8	Jamal	Science Club – noise from air conditioner	☐ I ☑ D ☐ N
10/8	Danni	Reading area – lights in classroom too bright	☐ I ☑ D ☐ N
10/15	Jamal	Science Club – noise from air conditioner	☐ I ☐ D ☑ N
10/21	Amelie	Cafeteria – too hot	☑ I ☐ D ☐ N

SOS Strategy Data Collection

Figure 2.14. SOS strategy data collection tool–example.

Planning and Organizing: *Environmental Checklist Strategy*

Checklists have been used in many different environments to provide the necessary steps in a process or to organize tasks. In healthcare and aviation, the use of checklists has been credited with a reduction in spending, injury, and loss of life (Gawande, 2009). For students with ASD, a checklist can work as a memory aid, and can provide information for the student regarding *what* tasks need to be completed, *how much* needs to be done, and *when* the task is finished (Aspy & Grossman, 2012; Wilkins & Burmeister, 2015).

An environmental checklist can be used to *analyze* the current environment, based on specific criteria, *identify* any needed changes, and *document* when changes have been made. A checklist that clarifies environmental attributes can be used independently by the student in new environments to proactively identify any trouble areas, and initiate a problem-solving strategy to deal with the problem (see PLACE in the next section).

 Why Is This Important?

The function of the environmental checklist is to support the student by analyzing and identifying those environmental characteristics that lead to greater productivity and less stress. The goal of the checklist is to increase the student's awareness of environmental conditions that are conducive to a positive work environment, whether at school, at work, or at home.

Teachers: When and How to Use a Checklist

Use the *Classroom Environment Checklist* (see Figure 2.15, Appendix A) to identify areas within the classroom that may be potential trouble areas for students. Develop a plan to fix any items on the checklist that are rated "no" or "partial."

Stage 1 Learners

For Stage One learners, collect data on individual students, using the *Student Environmental Preference Checklist* (see Figure 2.16, Appendix A) to determine individual student preferences. Make changes as needed for individual students. An example of the *Classroom Environment Checklist* (see Figure 2.15) shows how Ms. Rosales conducted a pre-assessment of her classroom environment indicating a number of areas to improve.

Stage 2 Learners

For Stage Two learners, interview the student, using the items on the *Student Environmental Preference Checklist* (see Figure 2.16, Appendix A) to guide the process. Share your thoughts with the student regarding elements of the environment. Discuss ways that elements within the environment might be changed to meet the student's needs. Note those areas that are most important for the student's comfort and productivity.

For Stage Three learners, have the student use the checklist independently in a variety of different environments. Discuss possible changes or adaptations (such as wearing headphones in a noisy environment) that could be made to improve an environment and make it more acceptable (see *Directions for Students* below).

Directions for Students

When and How to Use a Checklist

- It's important to know what things in the environment help you learn.
- You can use the *Student Environmental Preference Checklist* (see Figure 2.16 in Appendix A) to decide what helps the most. You can also use the checklist to evaluate a new environment and to figure out if you might need to change some things to be successful.
- If there are things in a new environment that are not helpful, are there things you can change? Use the checklist to identify any trouble spots and then work with a teacher, supervisor, or another adult to identify ways the environment might be changed to meet your needs. You may choose to use the PLACE process (see the section on Problem Solving in this chapter) to help you solve the problem of an environment that does not meet your needs.

Classroom Environment Checklist			

Teacher Name: _____Ms. Rosales_____ Date: _____10/23_____

☑ Pre-assessment ☐ Post-assessment

Environmental Component	Yes	No	Partial
1. Individualization and personal connection: Students are given ways to build ownership and a personal connection to the classroom through a display of personal work and interests. Notes: _Student work displayed. Need to incorporate interests (Pokemon?)._			X
2. Adaptability and flexibility: The classroom design is flexible enough to allow a variety of activities *or* the design can be changed easily to accommodate different activities. Notes: _Science center._			X
3. Color and contrast: The classroom has a good balance of color and is neither too colorful nor too bland. Notes: _None_	X		
4. Visual stimulation: The classroom offers some visual stimulation, but it is not overwhelming. No more than 80% of the wall space is covered. Notes: _Probably need to reduce displays._		X	
5. Lighting: The classroom is well lit and uses primarily natural light, augmented by electric light. If fluorescent light is primarily used, there are areas in the classroom lit by alternate means. Notes: _The fluorescent lights are bright & make humming noise._		X	
6. Air quality: There is appropriate circulation of air in the room. Notes: _Can be stuffy in summer._		X	
7. Temperature: The temperature is neither too warm nor too cold. Notes: _Too hot in summer. Get fan._		X	
8. Use of space and organization: The classroom is well organized and uncluttered. The teacher is able to monitor all areas of the room. Notes: _All areas/bins labeled._	X		
9. Sound: Classroom noise is minimized through the use of carpet or padded bottoms on chairs and tables. There is no discernable noise from the air conditioner or lighting. Notes: _Lights hum, announcements from office can be distracting._		X	
10. Safe place: There is a safe place available for students to access. This space is designed to provide a sensory break and has fidgets and other items available. Notes: _Classroom library has bean bag chairs and hand fidgets available._	X		
Totals	3	5	2

Figure 2.15. Classroom environmental preference checklist–example.

Student Environmental Preference Checklist			
Student Name: _____ Desiray _____			
Date: _____ 10/24 _____			
Data collector: _____ Ms. Rosales _____			
Role: _____ Teacher _____			
☑ Pre-assessment ☐ Post-assessment			
Environmental Component	**Yes**	**No**	**Partial**
1. Color and contrast: Colors are neither too bright nor too dull, and are nice to look at. Notes: _I don't like the ugly brown walls._		x	
2. Visual stimulation: The walls in the classroom are not too crowded with stuff. Notes: _I like the art bulletin board._	x		
3. Lighting: The lights in the classroom do not bother me. They are not too bright or too noisy. Notes: _The lights hurt my eyes._		x	
4. Air quality: The room smells OK and is not too stuffy. Notes: _Smells fine._	x		
5. Temperature: The temperature isn't too warm or too cold. Notes: _Too hot._		x	
6. Use of space and organization: The classroom looks organized and neat. Notes: _It's nice._	x		
7. Noise Level: The classroom is usually quiet, and there are no noises that bother me. Notes: _The loudspeaker for morning announcements is too loud._		x	
Totals	3	4	0

Figure 2.16. Student environmental preference checklist–example.

Data Collection:

The *Student Environmental Preference Checklist* can be used as a pre-assessment and post-assessment to identify needed areas for change, and how those changes have been made (see Figure 2.16, Appendix A). In the example checklist (see Figure 2.16), Desiray's answers show four areas in the classroom environment that are not effective for her, giving the teacher ideas for making improvements in the classroom. Once Desiray has had time to experience the changes in the environment, the teacher can use the *Student Environmental Preference Checklist* to collect post-assessment data.

Problem Solving: *PLACE Strategy*

It was the first day of school and Lettie loved her 4ᵗʰ grade class! Her best friend was in her class, and her new teacher, Ms. Mills, was really nice. After the first week of school, Lettie started to get a stomachache every day before math at 11:00, and she had a hard time paying attention. By Thursday of the second week, she felt sick as soon as she arrived at school and asked to go to the nurse. She also did not have her math homework because she hadn't been able to pay attention and didn't know what to do.

On Friday, Ms. Mills talked to her after reading and asked if she was feeling OK. Lettie started to cry and said she felt sick. Lettie told her teacher that she started to feel sick every day after morning group, when each table of students took turns to add a word for the day to the Word Wall. Ms. Mills was concerned and decided to implement a strategy to help Lettie discover what was causing her to feel sick, and then work through a solution to allow her to participate in class and complete her work.

For students with autism, well-structured and predictable environments lead to greater success academically, socially, and behaviorally. When difficulties related to the classroom environment occur, the *PLACE Strategy* can be used in teaching students how to problem solve.

It is applicable to students of all ages and can be used in classroom settings across the school campus. The PLACE card (see Figure 2.17) can be used as a visual support to define the process by answering the following five questions:

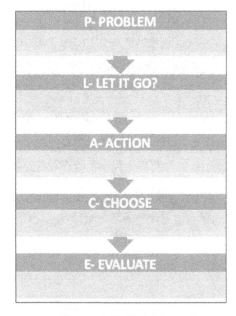

1. **P** Is there a **P**roblem in my environment?
2. **L** **L**et it go? If no, next step.
3. **A** What are some **A**ctions?
4. **C** Which action will I **C**hoose?
5. **E** **E**valuate- Did this work for me?

Responses will vary based on student perceptions of the problem, as well as individual student needs. In the example about Lettie, Ms. Mills implemented the steps for the *PLACE Strategy* and helped Lettie determine that she did have a <u>Problem</u>. As they talked about what happened in the morning, Ms. Mills discovered

Figure 2.17. PLACE card.

that Lettie was getting bumped by all of the students who walked past to her to get to the activity table. Ms. Mills asked Lettie if this was a problem she could "<u>Let go.</u>" Lettie said it made her feel nervous (anxious) and scared (dysregulated) each morning. They decided this was not something Lettie could let go. Ms. Mills guided Lettie to consider two "<u>Actions</u>" or ideas to solve the problem. The first action idea was to move to a different table away from the traffic area. Another was to sit in a different seat at her table. Lettie chose to sit in a different seat at her table because she wanted to stay with her friends. Ms. Mills and Lettie decided to check in after one week to see how things were going. At that time Lettie could <u>Evaluate</u> how this strategy had worked for her.

Why Is This Important?

The function of PLACE is to help the student analyze a problem related to the environment, determine a solution, and respond appropriately. The goal is for the student to be an active decision maker in determining strategies that allow him to succeed in typical as well as unpredictable environments.

Teacher Directions: When and How to Use PLACE

The *Environmental Problem-Solving Chart* will guide the student through the process, as shown in the examples on the chart below (see Figure 2.18). This should start as a structured lesson using familiar examples students can understand or have experienced. Move on to using actual problems as they occur in classroom or campus environments. Once students are familiar with PLACE, use it as a preventative strategy.

Directions for Students

When and How to Use PLACE

You can use the PLACE process independently when you feel challenged by situations in the school environment. Choose a place to keep the PLACE card such as:

- o in your reminder binder or a folder in your backpack,
- o on your electronic device,
- o in a spot in your class or other place with easy access.

When you feel stressed or anxious because of something negative about the environment, use the *PLACE Strategy* by answering the questions on the card. You can write your answers on the *Environmental Problem-Solving Chart* (see Figure 2.19, Appendix A) or just think it through.

After you use the strategy, it's a good idea to debrief with your teacher so you both are aware of the problem and the actions that solve the problem for you.

Environmental Problem Solving Chart Examples				
Problem	**Let it go?**	**Actions**	**Choose**	**Evaluate**
Examples: • Getting bumped when in a group in class or on campus • Sun is too bright coming through the windows • Lights have loud buzz in class, cafeteria, library • Assigned to a table with four students; we are touching and it's crowded • Students bump into my chair on their way to pencil sharpener or sink • When lining up, students shove and bump into me • Sitting under vent and air blows directly on me • Difficulty sitting at my desk for an entire work period	If it is a little problem, can I ignore it or find a solution on my own? If it is a big problem, • Who can I go to for help (teacher, lunch proctor, para-professional, etc.)? • What actions can I take, or what do I need to do next?	Some options: • Move to a different desk or table group • Use headphones • Use a fidget • Go to my "safe place" for a few minutes (e.g., a designated area which could be a section of the classroom, a support provider's office, or another location on campus where an adult is present) • Go to the end of the line to keep from getting bumped • Use flexible seating, e.g., add a stability disc to my chair or use a therapy ball • Use a portable 3-sided privacy screen at my desk	Which actions can I choose to take? What action is the best choice for me?	<u>Before</u>: How will I know that I made the right choice of an action? <u>During</u>: How am I feeling? If I'm feeling that there is still a problem, what other action can I take? <u>After</u>: How did the actions I chose work? Did they solve the problem? What can I do differently next time?

Figure 2.18. PLACE strategy sample environmental problem-solving chart.

Reproduce the PLACE card (see Figure 2.17) as appropriate to the student's needs and abilities, such as:

- Copy on 9" by 11" paper (allowing student to write responses directly on the card).
- On an index card or business card (a portable and discreet visual reminder of the steps).
- Store the PLACE card steps on an electronic device.

Stage 1 Learners

For Stage One learners, use the *PLACE Environmental Problem Solving Chart* (see Figure 2.19, Appendix A) to introduce the PLACE process to the student. First, show him the PLACE card and go over each prompt. Directly teach, reinforce, practice, and reteach each step of the process until the student can go through the steps using the PLACE card with minimal support.

Stage 2 Learners

For Stage Two learners, create stories and role-plays in which you model the steps to solve a problem (see Figure 2.18 examples) using a "think-aloud" process. Next, have students work in pairs to practice, using examples of problem situations and brainstorming answers for the PLACE card. Be ready to remind the student to use PLACE when you see they are being challenged by environmental problems in the classroom, on campus, or in other environments.

Stage 3 Learners

For Stage Three learners, as the student becomes proficient at using the process, gradually release responsibility so that the process ultimately shifts from teacher-directed to student-directed (see *Directions for Students* below).

All Learners

For learners in all stages, promote generalization by encouraging students to recall environmental problems in other settings and what actions have been effective.

PLACE Environmental Problem-Solving Chart				
Student: Lettie Teacher: Ms. Mills				
Date: 10/24				
Problem	**Let it go?**	**Actions**	**Choose**	**Evaluate**
I sit at a table with four other students who talk a lot and are loud. They also bump and touch me when moving to and from the table.	I get very frustrated with my table partners and could lose control and yell or even hit the other students when they keep talking. It is a big problem for me and I can't ignore it. I need to talk to the teacher about what I can do about the problem.	I have three options: Move to a different desk or table group. Take breaks in the back of the room for five minutes when I feel overwhelmed. Wear headphones.	My choice is Action #2- to stay with the group and take breaks when I feel overwhelmed from the talking and bumping.	Before: I wanted to stay with this group because I like them and another group might not be better. During: I will keep track of how many breaks I needs to take. After: I feel this solved the problem. I was a little worried about missing activities during my breaks.

Figure 2.19. PLACE environmental problem-solving chart used by student and/or teacher–example.

Data Collection

Once the student has an action plan to solve the problem, the teacher can use the *PLACE Data Collection Chart* (see Figure 2.20, Appendix A) to record how the student uses the *PLACE Strategy*. In the following example, Ms. Mills assessed Lettie's use of PLACE noting that she followed the first four steps independently and needed reminders and prompts for the last step (see Figure 2.20).

PLACE Teacher Data Collection				
Student: Lettie Teacher: Ms. Mills				
Date: 10/24				
Student completed each step: **Independently = I** **or with Prompts = P**				
Problem	**Let it go?**	**Actions**	**Choose**	**Evaluate**
☑ I ☐ P	☑ I ☐ P	☐ I ☑ P	☑ I ☐ P	☐ I ☑ P
Comments: Described the problem.	**Comments:** Knew she couldn't let it go.	**Comments:** Needed help with possible actions.	**Comments:** Made her own choice.	**Comments:** Needed reminders and prompts to use the action (take break) and to evaluate.

Figure 2.20. PLACE teacher data collection tool–example.

CHAPTER 3

STRUCTURING CLASSROOM TIME TO MAXIMIZE STUDENT LEARNING

Jack started high school and soon became involved in multiple extracurricular activities. Before he knew it, winter break was on the horizon, and with that came the end of the trimester. With reports due, as well as having to study for final exams, Jack found that he had not considered his workload and, as a result, had not managed his time well in balancing his academic needs with his other activities. Recognizing that Jack was at risk of failing some of his classes, his teachers met to discuss their concerns. They felt that Jack would be a good candidate for the school site's intervention class, a program that was staffed by special educators, as well as general education teachers, and designed to provide short-term extra support for any student at risk of not promoting to the next grade. It was suggested that Jack attend the program twice a week in place of his P.E. class.

Jack was able to get one-on-one help from the teacher in the intervention class. One of the first things she did was to look at Jack's planning system. Like all students at school, he was provided with a planner to keep track of assignments. Jack, who had fine motor deficits that made hand-writing a significant challenge, was using a laptop and submitting assignments in a digital format, but he was not doing a good job of keeping track of assignments and due dates in the planner, as that required him to write the information.

The intervention class teacher suggested that Jack use a Google Calendar, and taught him how to use many of its features, including those that encouraged estimating the time needed for tasks and projects in order to meet deadlines. Jack attended his intervention class for six weeks, receiving support in priority setting and time management, and was soon capable of budgeting his time more productively and meeting deadlines at school.

Some of the most important components of structuring effective classrooms include establishing and teaching typical routines and procedures and incorporating strategies to teach students how to manage time. Teaching time management from the early grades through high school can be effective in helping students be good time managers in adulthood. This chapter will highlight the importance of structuring classroom time, developing routines, and teaching time management strategies in a way that builds executive function skills. You and your students will learn four strategies. For each of these strategies, you will learn steps to gradually shift responsibility to the student, so that the student acquires the ability to self-organize, in order to eventually plan and monitor multiple activities as an adult. Blank copies of all of the tools in this chapter are also provided in Appendix B.

Link to Executive Function

Structuring classroom time by developing and teaching classroom routines, using visual schedules, and supporting students in planning, prioritizing, and completing assignments increases structure and predictability, decreases anxiety, and provides opportunities for students to engage in activities with greater independence, which supports academic and behavioral success. Table 3.1 shows the connection between structuring time, time management, and EF skills.

Structuring Classroom Time and Evidence-Based Practices

A number of evidence-based practices support using classroom structure, routines, and time management strategies. Classrooms with consistent routines facilitate student understanding of expectations in the learning environment (Ostrosky, Jung, Hemmeter, & Thomas, 2008). A number of evidence-based practices support using classroom structure, routines, and time-management strategies described in this chapter. Successful implementation of routines incorporates a task analysis, the breaking down of complex behavioral skills into smaller components, explicitly teaches routines, and can be used proactively

EBPs in this Chapter
• Task Analysis
• Antecedent-Based Intervention
• Visual Supports
• Self-Management
• Reinforcement
• Video Modeling

as an antecedent-based intervention. These routines then act to reduce challenging behavior during less structured times, as well as infrequent events (Kern & Clemmons, 2007). Individualized visual schedules can reduce challenging behavior by limiting the impact of various events (e.g., stressful activities, unpredictable transitions) (O'Reilly, Sigafoos, Lancioni, Edrisinha, & Andrews, 2005). Visual schedules help structure classroom time and clearly articulate expectations in a visual format, allowing students to develop an understanding of time, anticipate upcoming events and activities, make transitions, manage anxiety, develop flexibility, and become as independent as possible.

Visual schedules are an evidence-based practice within the category of visual supports (Wong et al., 2014) and schedules (National Autism Center, 2015). Routines and schedules can be put into place as part of an effective time management system, supporting the self-management skill of helping students manage their own routines and schedules independently (DiPipi-Hoy & Steere, 2016). Finally, combining all of these techniques with reinforcement, another evidence-based practice, can strengthen the behaviors necessary for initiation and independent follow-through on activities.

Link to Executive Function Skills			
Areas of Executive Function	**Structuring classroom time and routines provides support by:**	**Adults who have learned these skills will be able to:**	**Real-world examples of effective EF skills:**
Developing flexibility	Giving students predictable procedures and routines so that they can move smoothly from one activity to the next without losing learning time.	Adapt to changes and be effective time managers for successful employment, postsecondary education, vocational, home, leisure, and community activities.	Uses a personal calendar and updates it on a regular basis. Adjusts to a rotating schedule at work. Develops a timeline to get a job done.
Leveling emotions	Assisting students in managing anxiety and distress over school activities.	Use self-regulation strategies to manage anxiety and distress when there are changes in routines and schedules.	Itemizes and prioritizes tasks. Strategically uses sticky notes as visual reminders.
Increasing impulse control	Providing structure around expectations about the classroom systems.	Organize time with visual reminders and alternate preferred and non-preferred tasks to decrease distractions and increase likelihood for completing tasks.	Customizes schedule to reflect choices, and makes plans in advance to reduce distractions and impulsive behavior to complete tasks on time.
Planning and organizing	Making classroom systems transparent and supporting students in personal planning and organization.	Organize events of a day/week/month/year on a personal schedule and manage one's schedule and tasks effectively.	Chunks tasks and projects to stay organized, and sets deadlines to stay on track.
Problem solving	Communicating expectations and the "why" behind those expectations, so that students can become more actively involved in problem solving, initially with support, and independently in the future.	Recognize when there is a problem with completing tasks or managing time, and brainstorm possible solutions, then select and implement a solution.	Adapts to changes in a task by adjusting the work to meet new requirements or due dates. Prioritizes tasks around a timeline. Uses steps to effectively solve problems as they come up.

Table 3.1. Link between EF skills and structuring classroom time.

Flexibility: Time Management Strategies

Being able to manage time, which includes being aware of one's use of time and being able to manage one's schedule and tasks effectively (Wilkins & Burmeister, 2015), is an important life skill. Although the concept of time may seem abstract, many students with EF deficits learn how to successfully *tell* time, but without explicit instruction they may not be able to develop effective time management, a skill that supports and builds flexibility. Students benefit when teachers clearly integrate time management skills that are implied in academic standards into the curriculum at all grade levels.

 Why Is This Important?

Effective time management can help a student set priorities, complete assignments on time, and plan for the future. Students can increase their independence in daily living and adaptive skills through learning to regulate their use of time. Viewing time management as an important step toward independence and explicitly teaching the behaviors that support our students in becoming effective time managers can potentially increase an individual's quality of life (DiPipi-Hoy & Steere, 2016).

Teacher Directions: When and How to Teach Time Management

Time management starts with an awareness of time in daily routines and activities. Students develop an understanding of the passage of time through participating in activities with clear start and end times. Students must also be able to estimate the time needed to complete school assignments or tasks within a requisite time frame, which supports learning to set priorities, an important step towards effective time management (Wilkins & Burmeister 2015).

Stage 1 Learners Stage One learners learn the steps to estimate, predict, and compare time predictions through modeling, support, practice, and reinforcement by using the activities shown in *Estimating Time* (Figure 3.1.). List familiar routines/ activities in the day, then ask students to estimate which activity will take longer to complete. Next, ask students to predict how long it will take to complete specific daily activities. Finally, ask students to compare their estimate/prediction with the actual time it took to complete the activity.

Stage 2 Learners Stage Two learners can learn time management skills by taking turns as "Time Leaders" during group or classroom activities, as shown on the *Time Awareness and Measurement* table (see Table 3.2).

Stage 3 Learners Stage Three learners work as "Time Managers" to independently manage their own time. Guide, prompt and reinforce these students, so they can independently perform the skills shown in *Time Awareness and Measurement* (see Table 3.2.). (See *Directions for Students* below.)

Estimating Time

Estimate
Name two of your daily routines/activities. Which one takes longer to complete? Think about activities such as getting ready for school, eating lunch, dressing for PE.

Predict
How long do you think it will take to complete common activities? Think about activities such as walking to the cafeteria, reading a chapter in a book, defining vocabulary.

Compare
What do you learn when you compare times for completing different activities? Complete the activity and compare your prediction or estimate to the actual time to complete the task.

Figure 3.1. Estimating time–steps for learning time estimation.

Time Awareness and Measurement		
Activities & Tools	**Stage 2: Time Leader Role**	**Stage 3: Time Manager Role**
Use a class calendar to increase awareness of activities and events.	Adds information and events to the classroom calendar. All students then add these to their personal calendars.	Uses a personal calendar (paper or electronic) and updates on a daily basis to add events, assignments, and activities.
Use various types of clocks to understand the passage of time.	Uses their personal watch or a classroom clock to report time to the class for transitions.	Keeps track of time using their watch, device, or a clock to initiate transitions to activities.
Use a structured schedule that chunks activities to understand passage of time.	Shows the order of activities on the class calendar and then on a personal schedule or calendar (use schedule cards or write as a list).	Writes own schedule and marks off each activity when completed.
Use a visual schedule of activities to understand units of time.	Visually shows the start and end times for classroom activities by writing the times on the board or using visual supports (e.g., start/end time cards).	Sets the start and end time for their assignments and activities using their personal timer (watch, device, wind-up timer).
Use timers to understand the length or unit of time for activities.	Sets the start and end times for classroom activities using the classroom timer.	Uses a personal timer (watch, device, wind-up timer) and sets their own time for events, assignments, and activities.

Table 3.2. Time awareness and measurement activities and roles.

All Learners

Teach and reinforce time management skills using student-friendly time management tools (see *Directions for Students below*). A variety of tools are specifically created to help students understand and practice time management. Consider low technology--such as clocks, timers, watches, and calendars--to organize time and provide reminders. Higher-tech devices can be programmed to give auditory, visual, or kinesthetic reminders linked to either time or location and may include:

- **Timers** that provide a visual and/or auditory signal, indicating when the time for an activity has ended. The Time Timer® is one of the most popular visual timers, available in several sizes or as an app.
- **Digital calendars** or calendar apps that provide schedules and reminders linked to specific alarms (e.g., set an alarm every Wednesday to sign and turn in time card).
- **Smart watches** have many options with simple or complex alarms for single or multiple activities. Smart watches are a popular choice as these devices can do almost everything that smartphones or tablets can do, but are smaller and more portable.
- **Smartphones and tablets** with apps for any task, from scheduling to keeping data and records regarding school assignments, hobbies, health, etc.
- Artificial intelligence **voice-activated devices** are interactive and can be easily programmed verbally to give reminders, make calls, and provide companionship. Voice-activated artificial intelligence devices such as Alexa and Siri can control everything from prompts, reminders to complete a task, and alarms to take medication. Voice-activated devices can also provide instant and almost unlimited information and resources with a simple verbal request.

Directions for Students

How You Can Be Your Own Time Manager

Learning to manage time is an important skill that helps you be successful in life. Here are some things to do to manage your time:

1. Use a schedule. Choose the best way to keep a schedule, such as:
   a. Write your schedule on a calendar or in a schedule book.
   b. Put your schedule into your device (phone, tablet, watch) by typing into a calendar app.
   c. If you have a voice-activated device (Alexa, Siri, etc.), you can tell your device to add activities to your calendar.
2. Use a reminder system. Choose the best way to get reminders such as:
   a. Check and read the activities on your calendar the night before, at the beginning of the day, and during the day.
   d. Put alarms into your device to remind you of important activities and deadlines.
   e. Make reminder lists for activities with lots of steps, such as getting ready in the morning, making dinner, doing laundry, paying bills, etc.

Remember, managing your time successfully is one of the most important skills to have as an adult.

Data Collection

Use the *Task Checklist Time Progress Monitoring* form below (see Figure 3.2, Appendix B) to monitor progress on a student's ability to get tasks done on time. In the example below, Jack did not get his tasks done on time as he started his day but was able to get to English and Science class on time (Figure 3.2). This information can be used to determine how to support Jack as he works on time management.

Task Checklist Time Progress Monitoring			
Name: Jack		Date: 11/10	
1. List the time and tasks or activities to be completed. 2. Did the student complete the task or activity on time? Check yes or no.			
Time to Complete	**Activity**	**Completed on Time?**	
8:15	Turn in homework, get out supplies	☐ Yes	☑ No
8:25	Complete journal paragraph	☐ Yes	☑ No
8:45	Dress for PE and line up for class	☐ Yes	☑ No
9:45	Change, go to English class, have materials ready	☑ Yes	☐ No
10:45	Take break and go to Science class by the bell	☑ Yes	☐ No

Figure 3.2. Task checklist time progress monitoring data collection form–example.

Leveled Emotionality: Strategies for Using Visual Schedules

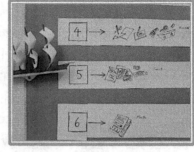

Collin had a difficult time following verbal directions, especially when making transitions from one activity to the next throughout the school day in his 8th grade class. He appeared highly anxious, argued with the adults in the classroom, and often struggled to regulate his emotions, resulting in what his teacher called a "meltdown." A functional behavior assessment (FBA) was conducted in partnership with Collin's parents and school staff to identify circumstances and consequences

Figure 3.3. Visual schedule with Collin's special interest area.

associated with his disruptive behaviors. The FBA identified the antecedent as difficulties in transitioning from one activity to another, resulting in an IEP goal related to making successful transitions. His team decided to implement an individual schedule to help Collin make sense of his day. Assessment indicated that a full-day schedule, using a combination of text and pictures, would best support Collin in developing an understanding of time, anticipating upcoming events and activities, and ultimately making successful transitions.

Everyone on the team knew how much Collin loved ships and incorporated this special interest into his individual visual schedule (see Figure 3.3). With direct instruction and consistency, Collin learned how to follow the schedule by moving a ship from one activity to the next. It didn't take long before Collin was successfully navigating his way throughout his day (see Figure 3.4). Data indicated that use of his schedule produced a dramatic decrease in disruptive behaviors during transitions. At his IEP at the end of the year, his team revised his schedule to a less obvious and more portable check-off system that would provide support in his high school classes and activities (see Figure 3.5).

Figure 3.4. Using the schedule.

Collin's Schedule

_____ Journal

_____ Spelling

_____ Reading

_____ Recess

_____ Math

_____ Lunch

_____ P.E.

_____ Choice Activity

_____ Bus

Figure 3.5. Collin's notebook schedule.

Many of us use a calendar as a visual tool to stay organized. Scheduling events and activities on a calendar establishes a predictable routine and provides a well-defined external structure that can tell us where we should be, what we should be doing, and when we should be there. Students with autism often experience high anxiety due to unexpected changes, so increasing a student's flexibility and ability to regulate his emotions by using structure can help him become calmer and more independent. Whether a schedule is on a paper calendar, in a daily planner, or on an electronic device, schedules are tools that help all of us structure our time, use that time appropriately, and remain calm while accomplishing our daily routines. While routines represent procedures or practices, schedules represent the big picture – the activities to be completed daily or within a specific school setting (Ostrosky et al., 2008).

For students with autism, concepts related to time are abstract and can be difficult. An individual student schedule is a visual support used to structure and manage time and is a highly effective evidence-based practice (Wong, et. al, 2014). Whether students receive their educational services in special education or general education settings, visual schedules are applicable to many skill domains and can be used across settings. Schedules can be tailored to accommodate a variety of types of individuals. Their use is not limited to a particular age range, diagnosis, or level of cognitive functioning (Koyama & Wang, 2011). As a student uses her schedule independently, it becomes a self-management tool, allowing her to complete tasks on her own at school, at home, at work, and in the community.

 ## Why Is This Important?

Individual visual schedules provide students with visual information about where they are supposed to be and what they should be doing at a given time. Schedules help teach the importance of organization in a day, help teach the concept of discrete events, assist in developing sequential memory, and help a student understand the order in which activities will occur. Using visual schedules is an important way to provide the student with predictability and can help staff teach students to be flexible and use appropriate coping strategies when there is a change in schedule.

The scenarios on the following pages illustrate how implementation of an individual schedule helps structure daily classroom time and assists students in developing executive function skills by improving their flexibility and ability to self-regulate, thereby increasing their academic and social success.

Allan. *After receiving his educational services in a special education class, Allan was excited to be integrated with his peers in a general education elementary classroom. He had successfully used various schedule formats, starting with an object schedule in kindergarten, progressing to a picture schedule that was set up in the transition area of his special education classroom, and then moving to a written check-off schedule that he kept on a mini clipboard attached to the side of his desk with a hook & loop fastener. Data collection indicated that he was successful at using this written check-off schedule, so when Allan transitioned to the general education setting, his schedule went with him (see Figure 3.6).*

Written Check-Off Schedule
Sample

Name: *Allan*		Week Of: *Feb 13*

Today is: Monday   Tuesday   Wednesday   Thursday   (Friday)

✓	Activity	Comments
✓	Breakfast	*Say good morning to teachers and friends.*
✓	Seat work DOL	*Get folder and sit at desk, finish one page.*
✓	PE	*Change clothes.*
	Class Meeting	*Make 1 positive comment.*
	Language Arts	*Folder Activity #5: _____ Match Opposites.*
	Silent Reading	*Choose a book, read for 15 minutes.*
	Break	*Music or computer.*
	Math	*First listen to teacher and answer questions - then use calculator for Worksheet #_____.*
	Class Meeting	*Provide the weather forecast for tomorrow.*
	Lunch	*Choose healthy food.*
	Social Studies	*Work on group project.*
	Art	*Computer graphics.*
	Science	*Participate in magnet lesson by holding magnets and demonstrating how magnets attract certain items.*
	Review Day	*Gather belongings, review assignments.*

Figure 3.6. Written check-off schedule.

Knowing the benefit of individual visual schedules for students who have difficulty with transitions, and understanding that Allan was concerned about using visual supports that would make him look different from the other students, Allan's new teacher had individual schedules duplicated for additional students. Each student, including Allan, kept schedules in the front of their reminder binders and referred to them as needed. Allan had a very successful year, and his teacher also noted that disruptive behavior from other students during transitions that year was greatly reduced!

Kashan. An example of using visual schedules to support appropriate behavior is described by a parent who found that visual schedules worked not only at school but also at home for her son, Kashan. *"Kashan is in fourth grade and did really well with a visual word schedule (see Figure 3.7) that was attached to a clipboard. He enjoyed putting a check mark next to each item when he had completed an activity. During the first few weeks of school, Kashan demonstrated some interfering behaviors when it was time to make the transition from the group meeting to independent work. Using an antecedent-based intervention strategy, staff adjusted his schedule to provide a preferred activity (computer) following the non-preferred activity (independent work).*

Kashan's Schedule
☐ Morning Job
☐ Group Meeting
☐ Independent Work
☐ Computer
☐ Snack
☐ Recess
☐ 1:1 Work with Teacher
☐ Speech-Language Therapy
☐ Lunch
☐ 1:1 Work with Paraeducator
☐ Bus

Figure 3.7. Kashan's schedule.

Kashan's interfering behaviors decreased significantly, and he was able to make the transition when it was time for an independent work session. At home, we found that using the same type of schedule worked to get Kashan ready for bed. He did not like to shower or brush his teeth. By setting up the Xbox with his favorite video game after shower and tooth brushing, we were able to have a peaceful evening. This was a welcome change after years of meltdowns at bedtime."

Reina. *Reina, a high school student, had a part-time job at a local department store, receiving support through a program that was designed to move students from school into a career. Her job was to return items from the "go-back" bins to their proper place in the store. Reina was easily distracted, often wandered away from her assigned work area, and would impulsively approach and talk to customers. As a result, Reina didn't get her work done on time.*

Reina's job coach was aware that Reina was interested in having her own personal business card. Working collaboratively, her job coach and her supervisor developed a visual schedule (see Figure 3.8) that clearly illustrated her responsibilities at work. Using a business card template, the schedule was printed onto a business card, with several copies duplicated on cardstock. The supervisor ensured that a copy would be available when Reina checked in to work. Reina enjoyed having her own business card/schedule and kept one in her pocket, referring to it once she entered her work area. Reina particularly liked her last job of the day, vacuuming the area where the "go back" bins were located. Once the schedule was visual and Reina could "see" her last task

Reina's Work Schedule
✓ Sort items by department
✓ Place any broken items in "Discard" bin
✓ Put clothes on hangers
✓ Return items to department
✓ Vacuum floor in work area

Figure 3.8. Reina's "business card" work schedule.

of the day, she was able to focus on her work, and curtailed her spontaneous interactions with customers. Soon, Reina was successfully following her schedule and completing her assigned tasks.

Teacher Directions: When and How to Use Visual Schedules

Visual schedules can be used throughout the day in any setting. Initially, the student may be prompted by an adult to use his schedule, with the goal of having the student use his schedule independently in all environments. Adults often need to teach the student the meaning and value of a schedule.

Students who need more support to follow a schedule and transition between activities should be explicitly taught how to use a schedule to make smooth transitions and to complete all of their work and activities throughout the school day. Some students will carry a portable schedule (paper or device) while other students with more intensive needs can be supported to use a visual schedule located in the classroom. For information on determining what type of schedule is appropriate and individualizing it to meet a specific student's needs, see Appendix B: Chapter 3, *Guide for Developing and Teaching Visual Schedules*.

For students new to using visual schedules, the teacher can model using her own schedule and prompt the students to use their schedule for transition to each activity. Once the student understands how to use the schedule, other evidence-based practices can support full independence. For example, video modeling can also be used to teach the student how to use his schedule in the initial stages, or as a reteaching tool. As students begin to have success with their schedules, using social narratives will strengthen their understanding of schedule use.

Stage 1 Learners For Stage One learners, introduce the process of using a schedule by modeling how it is used. Directly teach, reinforce, practice, and reteach each step of the process until the student uses a schedule with minimal support. Let the student know that although teachers try their best to stay on schedule, the schedule might change. If possible, the teacher will try to let him know ahead of time.

Stage 2 Learners For Stage Two learners, teach the student how to be flexible and respond appropriately to unanticipated events by incorporating change into the student's schedule. For example, include adaptations for unplanned change by incorporating a visual cue (see Figures 3.9, 3.10, and 3.11). This can be a sticky note, hand-drawn notation for change, or an icon to indicate a cancelled or new activity. Involve the student in developing his schedule. As the student becomes more effective at using his schedule, have the student assist in setting up his own schedule.

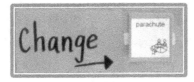

Figure 3.9. Visual cue for change in schedule.

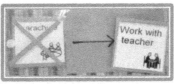

Figure 3.10. Visual cue for change to alternate activity.

Figure 3.11. Change attention signal or alert.

Stage 3 Learners

For Stage Three learners, support the student in developing his own schedule, gradually releasing responsibility so that the process ultimately shifts from a teacher-developed schedule to a student-developed schedule. As students become more independent in using their schedules, they may determine on their own when to check their schedules throughout the day (see *Directions for Students* below). Provide students with opportunities to collect data using the *Visual Schedules Progress Monitoring Form* (see Figure 3.12, Appendix B).

All Learners

For learners in all stages, encourage the students to use schedules in every setting to promote generalization. Train other teachers who support the student to promote generalization by also using schedules, so that schedules are used in all environments.

Directions for Students

When and How to Use a Visual Schedule

Use a visual schedule to help you organize your time and use your time appropriately. Your schedule should be based on your individual needs and can be in a variety of formats. You can use different types of schedules to meet your own needs. For example, you might use a schedule with photos or pictures, a written schedule, or a schedule on an electronic device. Choose the type of schedule that works best for you. Choose a place to keep your schedule, such as:

- in your classroom or someplace with easy access.
- in your reminder binder or folder in your backpack.
- on your electronic device.

Make sure you include the information on your schedule that helps you keep track of all of your activities. There will be activities that you are expected to have on your schedule, such as classes at school, but you may also add activities from outside of school, such as sports or doctor appointments. If you use a schedule in a daily planner or a digital app, you can put important events on your schedule, such as testing week or due dates for long-term assignments, so that you can plan ahead.

If you find that your schedule is not working to help you understand where you need to be and when you need to be there, ask one of your teachers or another adult for help.

Data Collection

Monitor progress by collecting data on a student's use of her visual schedule, including tracking the form of representation and the length of the schedule that the student uses (Sam & AFIRM Team, 2015). The *Visual Schedules Progress Monitoring Form* (see Figure 3.12, Appendix B) can be used to collect student data. If assessment data indicates that the student is not using a visual schedule appropriately, restructure and reteach, if needed. The *Visual Schedules Progress Monitoring*

Form example (Figure 3.12) shows Reina's progress over two weeks, as she became independent on most steps using her visual schedule.

Visual Schedules Progress Monitoring Form										
Student Name: Reina										
Indicate schedule details based on the Visual Assessment Tool:										
Form of schedule representation (pictures, symbols, words): words										
Length of schedule (half day, full day): full day (work day)										
Places schedule will be used (school, home, work): work										
Type of schedule (wall, folder, checklist, device): checklist										
Behavior	Date: 9/25	Date: 9/28	Date: 10/1	Date: 10/5	Date: 10/7	Date: 10/9	Date:	Date:	Date:	Date:
1. Initiates using schedule	P	P	I	I	I	I				
2. Follows schedule sequence	P	P	I	P	I	I				
3. Transitions to correct task/area	P	I	I	I	I	I				
4. Accepts changes with no advance warning	O	P	P	P	P	P				
Performance Key:	I = Independent				P = Prompt			O = No Response		
Notes: Reina needs support accepting changes with no advance warning. She likes using the schedule.										

Figure 3.12. Visual schedules progress monitoring form–example.

Impulse Control: *STARS Video Modeling Strategy*

Miss Swift, a new teacher fresh out of her university training program, was sharing some concerns with a seasoned fellow teacher, Ms. Gains. According to Miss Swift, her biggest behavioral challenges occurred during the first few minutes of the class period, when students entered her middle-school class and had to transition from "social" time in the school hallways as they traveled to the classroom, to "learning" time once they entered it. When Ms. Gains asked what her arrival routine was, Miss Swift responded that she hadn't given much thought to that when setting up her classroom. Ms. Gains suggested that she develop a routine for arrival time and teach the students what the behavioral expectations were for that routine.

Fresh from a staff development opportunity where she learned how to implement video modeling, Miss Swift decided to use that strategy to teach her students a morning arrival routine. She implemented video modeling to teach a routine, and within only two weeks' time Miss Swift reported to Ms. Gains that the difference in student behavior was amazing. She stated that students were now entering the classroom, putting their personal materials in the appropriate places, as well as any items that needed teacher attention, and starting the warm-up activities listed on the board. The students were then ready to focus when she called the class to order.

Routines play a significant role for students in school environments, helping them to understand what is expected of them throughout the day and providing them with cues for appropriate behaviors in those environments. For students with autism, routines provide comfort and ease (Pratt, 2014), helping them to calm down when they feel overwhelmed. Developing and implementing predictable routines maximizes structure and is a critical feature of effective classroom management (Simonsen & Fairbanks, n.d.).

When learning a new skill, many of us turn to videos as a visual model to show us the necessary steps, whether for changing a tire on a car, programming a new coffeemaker, or repairing an electronic device. Using video modeling is an evidence-based practice that provides a visual model of the behaviors (Wong, et.al, 2014), and can be an effective strategy to teach routines to students with autism. STARS is an acronym that outlines the steps for implementing video modeling, as shown in the *STARS Video Modeling Strategy* description (Figure 3.13).

 Why Is This Important?

Developing and teaching classroom routines increases structure and predictability, provides opportunities for students to engage in activities with greater independence, and supports student academic and behavioral success. Routines are especially important for students with autism, as routines can create stability and order, reducing anxiety by providing blueprints of expectations that render the environment more predictable and logical. Video modeling is an instructional technique that requires limited materials and teaches to the strengths of students with autism. As a visual tool, it can explicitly portray steps in a routine, is opportune for repetition, and is engaging for those who are motivated to learn through technology.

STARS Video Modeling Strategy	
★ S	**S**: **Select** the routine to teach/learn and the activity that will best demonstrate the routine. If using students in the video, use them to model only positive examples. If showing non-examples, use adults to demonstrate those behaviors.
★ T	**T**: **Task analyze** the steps for completing the specific routine by identifying the components or steps. (Simonsen et al., 2015).
★ A	**A**: **Analyze** baseline data. Are there parts of the routine that are more difficult than others?
★ R	**R**: **Record** the video. Decide in advance where, when, and how you will record the video. *Note:* If you are using students in the video clip, be sure to get parent permission.
★ S	**S**: **Show the video**. Plan when, how often, and where you will show the video, along with accompanying activities, such as class discussions.

Figure 3.13. STARS video modeling strategy.

Teachers: When and How to Use STARS to Teach Routines

Consider the role of routines throughout the school day and across settings, such as working in groups, working independently, getting materials, visiting the library, etc. Routines are especially important for less structured times such as transitions or free time, as well as less common events, such as emergency drills, field trips, or assemblies. Additional ideas include:

- Morning routine for starting the day or class (see examples in Figures 3.14 and 3.15)
- Completing morning work tasks
- Entering and exiting the classroom
- Listening to someone talk
- Asking a question
- Moving around the classroom
- Letting someone know you are sick
- Asking for something you need
- Getting homework after an absence
- Using "please" and "thank you"
- Packing up for the day

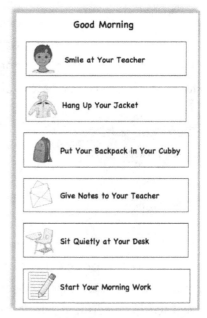

Figure 3.14. Elementary morning routine. Images ©LessonPix Inc. Used with permission.

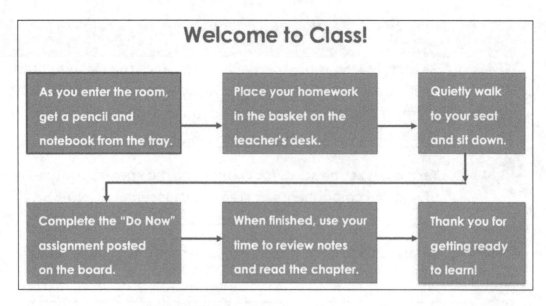

Figure 3.15. Secondary class start-up routine.

Stage 1 Learners For Stage One learners, introduce the idea of routines to the student. Point out examples of routines with which he may be familiar (e.g., the procedure for lining up with his class after the morning bell rings) and how they help students know and meet expectations. Use video modeling to directly teach the routine. Reinforce, practice, and reteach each step of the routine until the student can go through the routine with minimal support. Show the video often to reinforce expectations and post visual reminders of routines where students can see them. Prompt students to use the routine as an antecedent-based intervention. Additional evidence-based practices such as social narratives, modeling, prompting, and visual supports may be incorporated to assist with learning.

Stage 2 Learners For Stage Two learners, help the student develop flexibility by altering routines and periodically building in changes (Pratt, 2014). Reduce the use of the video as students become more capable of implementing the routine independently. Practice generalization of routines in different locations and at different times. Have students practice developing routines for different parts of the school day.

Stage 3 Learners For Stage Three learners, as the student becomes proficient at using the process, gradually release responsibility so that the process ultimately shifts from teacher-directed to student-directed (see *Directions for Students* below).

All Learners For learners in all stages, in addition to video modeling, consider incorporating visual supports to help clarify information regarding the routine and to communicate behavioral expectations. Such supports are based on students' needs and can be used with either the whole class or with individual students. Visual supports may be in the form of signs describing expectations for classroom procedures and routines, or on a card for individual students to refer to as needed. These signs or cards can be placed in strategic areas to remind students and staff how to accomplish daily tasks and activities.

Directions for Students

When and How You Can Use STARS to Learn a Routine

Learning a new routine can be hard. Sometimes a routine may be complicated, and you might forget some steps. Recording yourself or someone else completing the routine in a video can be a great way to learn the steps and practice them until you have mastered the entire routine. Making a video of a routine can be useful at school, at home, or at work. Other people may even find your video useful for learning the routine. Follow these steps to use STARS:

S - Select the routine you need to learn.
T - Task analyze the steps. Write down every necessary step in the routine.
A - Analyze the steps that may be most difficult. Plan how you'll record the video.
R - Record the video, starring you or someone else.
S - Study the video and use it to practice the steps..

Use these steps to make your own video, and then watch your STARS video to help you understand and learn a new routine.

 Data Collection

Routines are effective in maintaining order in the classroom and in teaching students how to function with more independence. Using video modeling can be an effective way to introduce and support student learning and mastery of routines. Collect data on student progress using the *Individual* or *Group Student Routine Data Collection Worksheets* (see Figures 3.16 & 3.17, Appendix B).

The first step in data collection for mastering routines is doing a task analysis of the desired routine. The distinct steps in the routine can be listed under the column titled "Individual Steps" as shown in the following examples–*Individual* (see Figure 3.16) or *Group* (see Figure 3.17) *Student Routine Data Collection Forms*. Once the individual steps have been identified, collect baseline data (A column) on each step, using the scoring key on the form.

After baseline data has been collected, provide instruction to the student by showing the video of the routine each day for one week. During this time, collect data on the student's performance of the steps in the B columns. During weeks two and three, collect data once each week and enter these data in the C columns. If the student does not complete the steps with 80% accuracy, show the video again and continue to collect data as needed until the student can perform the steps independently.

Individual Student Routine Data Collection Worksheet								

Student: Mia Green **Routine:** Getting Ready for Recess

Directions:

1. Task analyze routine with steps in first column.
2. Collect baseline data in Column A.
3. Show video daily and practice routine for 1 week; collect 3 data points in B columns.
4. During weeks 2 -4 collect data 1 time and enter data in C columns.
5. If scores fall below "8" in Column C, show video and practice routine.

Scoring Key:
2 = Independent
1 = Prompt Needed
0 = No Response

Individual Steps: Date:	A. 10/2	B. 10/6	B. 10/8	B. 10/10	C. 10/13	C. 10/15	C. 10/17
1. Freeze when lights blink	1	2	2	2	1	1	1
2. Put activities away	1	1	1	1	1	1	1
3. Stand in work area	0	1	2	2	2	2	2
4. Wait for signal	0	1	1	2	2	1	1
5. Walk to the yellow line	0	0	1	2	2	1	2
Mastery = 8 out of 10 points. Total:	2	5	7	9	8	6*	7*

Comments: * Showed video on 10/15-10/17 and practiced routine. Will continue to show video and practice routine on Mondays of each week until mastery is reached for 3 consecutive weeks.

Figure 3.16. Individual student routine data collection worksheet–example.

Group Routine Data Collection Worksheet							
# Students in Group: 5 Students			**Routine:** ELA Group Work				

Directions:
1. Task analyze routine with steps in first column.
2. Collect baseline data in Column A, counting the number of students who perform the step independently.
3. Show video daily and practice routine for 1 week; collect 3 data points in B columns by counting students as in Step 2.
4. During weeks 2 -4 collect data one time and enter data in C columns by counting students who perform the step independently.
5. Check data in each column. If scores fall below "80%," show video and practice routine.
6. Use the "Individual Student Routine Data Collection" for students who consistently struggle to perform the routine independently.

Scoring Key:

Count and record the number of students who complete the step independently.

Individual Steps: Date:	A. 10/2	B. 10/6	B. 10/8	B. 10/10	C. 10/13	C. 10/15	C. 10/17
1. Move to reading area on signal	4/5	4/5	5/5	5/5	4/5	5/5	4/5
2. Quiet & look at teacher in 15 seconds	3/5	3/5	4/5	4/5	4/5	4/5	3/5
3. Raise hand-wait until called on to talk	3/5	3/5	4/5	5/5	5/5	4/5	4/5
4. Move back to desk on signal	1/5	2/5	2/5	4/5	4/5	3/5	4/5
5. Start practice work in 15 seconds	1/5	1/5	2/5	3/5	3/5	3/5	3/5
Mastery = 80% Total:	12/25 48%	13/25 52%	17/25 68%	21/25 84%	20/25 80%	19/25 76%*	18/25 72%*

Comments: *Showed video on 10/15-10/17 and practiced routine. Will continue to show video and practice routine on Mondays of each week until mastery is reached for 3 consecutive weeks. Identify individual students who will need additional practice.

Figure 3.17. Group routine data collection worksheet–example.

Planning and Organizing: *MAP Strategy*

Aden felt sick and couldn't get out of bed to go to school. The semester ended in two weeks. He had not started his paper for history class, and still had to finish his project comparing two authors for his 11th grade English class. On top of that, he needed to study for his geometry and biology finals. His parents kept asking how he was doing, but he was afraid to tell them about all of the assignments and finals that were coming up. On top of everything, his counselor, Ms. Henry, sent an appointment slip for him to come to her office. He was feeling out of control and anxious, and didn't know what to do, but his mom made him get up and go to school. He felt terrible in History and English when his teachers reminded everyone about the assignments. But after his meeting with Ms. Henry, everything felt much more under control. She helped him develop a plan using

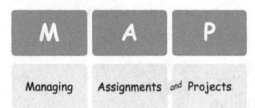

MAP (Manage Assignments and Projects) to get his paper and project done, and she found a study group to help him prepare for his finals. Aden was really glad he talked to Ms. Henry, and was happy that he now had the MAP strategy to help get all of his schoolwork organized and completed.

Students with autism are often at a loss when faced with a number of projects or assignments that need to be completed during the same time frame. These students often lack the skills to plan and organize their day to include schoolwork, leisure time, and home responsibilities. Planning requires students to anticipate future events in order to develop goals and steps to finish assignments and projects. Organizing requires the ability to use a system to keep track of the work completed, and to be completed in an organized manner (Freedman, 2010).

Students who have difficulty with planning and organizing often find it hard to complete projects, as they have no idea how to get started and lack the skills to make a plan and follow the steps needed to finish the project (Constable, Grossi, Moniz and Ryan, 2013). This inability to effectively plan and organize may increase stress and anxiety, causing additional behaviors that interfere with learning. A proactive strategy to assist students to plan and organize assignments and projects is MAP, an acronym that stands for **M**anage **A**ssignments and **P**rojects. The steps for using MAP are shown in Figure 3.18.

Steps for Using MAP
1. Identify the project assignment and the final due date.
2. Brainstorm the steps needed to complete the assignment, and use a calendar to find due dates for each step.
3. Write each action step on a sticky note with the due date in the top corner.
4. Place each sticky note on the MAP Graphic Organizer (GO) in the left column starting at the top with the steps that **need** to get done first.
5. Move tasks that are started and "in progress" to the middle column of the MAP GO.
6. As each task is completed– move it to the last column on the right side of the MAP GO. *The GOAL is to move each sticky note or step to the right side of the MAP Graphic Organizer!*
7. For multiple assignments, repeat steps 1-5 using a different colored sticky note and add to your GO as a visual reminder of tasks and due dates.

Figure 3.18. MAP–steps for using the manage assignments and projects strategy.

 ## Why Is This Important?

MAP gives students a set of steps for planning and organizing. This strategy can be used as a self-management tool to get assignments and projects done on time (Sam & Affirm Team, 2016b). The *MAP Graphic Organizer* (see Figure 3.19, Appendix B) is also an effective visual support when used in a portable format that the student can keep in his device or binder and use as a reminder of the steps for planning and organizing his assignments and projects (Sam & Affirm Team, 2015). With MAP, the student is in control of his work by planning and organizing his tasks and time, thereby allowing him to function successfully at school and at work. MAP can help students complete both a multi-step assignment such as a sixth-grade science fair project, as well as a set of assignments a college student with four classes would need to organize and turn in.

Teacher Directions: When and How to Use MAP

Teach the strategy as a structured lesson. Describe the meaning of the acronym for MAP, and use the *MAP Graphic Organizer* to describe the process by going over each step in the first section. Display the MAP GO as a poster and provide an individual printed copy for each student. The sample *MAP Graphic Organizer* (see Figure 3.19) illustrates how two assignments can be organized by using sticky notes to show each step and date for completion.

Stage 1 Learners For Stage One Learners, provide a poster version of the *MAP Graphic Organizer* (see Figure 3.19, Appendix B), along with a calendar and large sticky notes. Choose a class assignment that will last for three to four days as a way to model the MAP steps. Introduce the steps for MAP on the MAP GO and then model each of the steps for a class assignment, using the calendar and the large sticky notes to MAP it out on the MAP GO. Continue this process over three to four days. Have students participate by coming up to the MAP GO poster to move the sticky notes as tasks are completed.

Stage 2 Learners

For Stage Two Learners, the teacher continues to model three more class assignments on the *MAP Graphic Organizer* poster. For each assignment, students write tasks on sticky notes and then move the notes across their individual *MAP Graphic Organizers* as each task is completed.

Stage 3 Learners

For Stage Three Learners, students will use the *MAP Graphic Organizer* on their own as they become more proficient. The teacher should check in regularly to coach and reinforce the students (*see Directions for Students* below).

All Learners

For learners in all stages, to promote generalization, encourage the student to use the MAP GO is in other classes, especially mainstreaming, to promote generalization.

Directions for Students

When and How to Use MAP

You can use the *MAP Graphic Organizer* to plan and organize your assignments and projects when you have too much to do, and feel overwhelmed. Follow these steps for using MAP.

- Choose a place to keep the *MAP Graphic Organizer*, such as:
  o your binder or folder,
  o your computer or electronic device,
  o a spot in your class or other place with easy access.
- When you feel stressed because you have a lot of work to do, use the MAP GO (Figure 3.19 in Appendix B). Write each task and date on a sticky note, putting the sticky notes on the columns of the GO, and moving each note over until all the tasks are in the "Finished" column.

After you use the MAP, it's a good idea to debrief with your teacher so you both are aware of your assignments and projects. She can support you as you MAP out your steps and get everything done.

MAP: Managing Assignments *and* Projects Graphic Organizer
Student Name: Jack
1. Identify the project assignment and the final due date.
2. Brainstorm the steps needed to complete the assignment. Use a calendar to find due dates for each step.
3. Write each action step on a sticky note, with the due date in the top corner.
4. Place each sticky note on your *MAP Graphic Organizer* (GO) in the left column, starting at the top with the steps that **need** to get done first.
5. Move tasks that are started and in progress to the middle column of the MAP GO.
6. As each task is completed, move it to the last column on the right side of the MAP GO. *Your goal is to move each sticky note or step to the right side of the MAP GO!*
7. For multiple assignments, repeat steps 1-5 using a different colored sticky note, and add to your GO as a visual reminder of tasks and due dates.

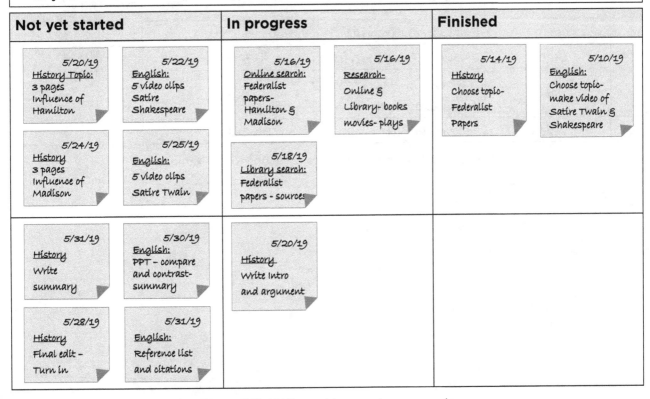

Not yet started	In progress	Finished
5/20/19 History Topic: 3 pages Influence of Hamilton 5/22/19 English: 5 video clips Satire Shakespeare	5/16/19 Online search: Federalist papers- Hamilton & Madison 5/16/19 Research- Online & Library- books movies- plays	5/14/19 History Choose topic- Federalist Papers 5/10/19 English: Choose topic- make video of Satire Twain & Shakespeare
5/24/19 History 3 pages Influence of Madison 5/25/19 English: 5 video clips Satire Twain	5/18/19 Library search: Federalist papers - sources	
5/31/19 History Write summary 5/30/19 English: PPT – compare and contrast- summary	5/20/19 History Write Intro and argument	
5/28/19 History Final edit – Turn in 5/31/19 English: Reference list and citations		

Figure 3.19. MAP graphic organizer–example.

Data Collection

Monitor progress by collecting data using the *MAP Data Collection* form (see Figure 3.20, Appendix B) to show if the *MAP Strategy* is successful, as evidenced by students completing assignments and projects on time. Data will include:

- The name of the target assignment or project.
- Number of steps needed to complete the assignment or project.
- Number of steps completed by the due dates.

If assessment data indicates students are not completing their assignments and projects on time, reteach the *MAP Strategy* and collect data to reassess. In the example below, Ms. Henry recorded data for two students showing their progress on English and History assignments (see Figure 3.20).

MAP Data Collection				
Start Date	Student Name	Name of Assignment or Project	Number of Assignment/ Project Steps	Number of Steps Completed by Due Dates
5/10	Jack	English- Satire Video	6 steps	4
5/10	Aden	English- Article Review	5 steps	3
5/14	Jack	History- Argument Paper	8 steps	5
5/14	Aden	History Project	9 steps	6

Figure 3.20. MAP classroom data collection form–example.

Problem Solving: *Get it Done Strategy*

Students with autism who lack competent EF skills may not work as independently on complex tasks and long-term projects as their typically developing peers. When presented with a multiple-step chore, large project, or assignment, students who have difficulty with problem solving may get frustrated with what seems like an insurmountable task. Even a one-page worksheet can cause a high level of anxiety. For these students, knowing they have a problem with getting their assignments completed is the first step in the *Get it Done Strategy*.

Subsequent steps guide the student to consider, choose and determine the effectiveness of one or more strategies, as shown in Figure 3.21 (see Appendix B for larger version). There are a variety of options that you can use to support students who struggle with starting and completing multi-step tasks and long-term projects. Providing a visual support, such as a template or graphic organizer to help organize content and ideas, is a useful tool.

Another option is to provide a worksheet related to the project that breaks down the assignment into component tasks or parts, with a clear description and due date for each part (see MAP Strategy).

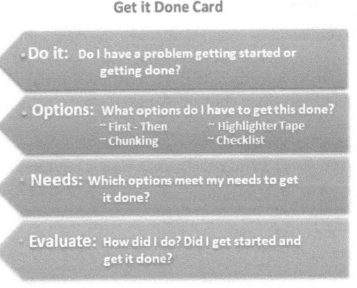

Get it Done Card

- **Do it:** Do I have a problem getting started or getting done?
- **Options:** What options do I have to get this done?
  ~ First - Then ~ Highlighter Tape
  ~ Chunking ~ Checklist
- **Needs:** Which options meet my needs to get it done?
- **Evaluate:** How did I do? Did I get started and get it done?

Figure 3.21. Get it done card template.

Allowing a student to complete the first one or two steps of a new task, rather than the whole assignment, is a curricular modification that provides students with supports they may need to participate as independently as possible (Neitzel, 2010). Four strategies in particular that can support students in reducing anxiety and frustration include *first-then cards, chunking folders, highlighter tape*, and *checklists*.

First-Then Cards

For a student who just can't seem to get started on an activity or assignment, or who has difficulty switching between activities, using a visual support in the form of a card that indicates first-then (see Figure 3.22) may be useful. This visual strategy can reduce anxiety and frustration by helping a student make a transition or simply get started on an activity, as well as supporting students in completing non-preferred tasks, by having the first task followed by something that is preferred (Browning Wright, 2011). Depending on the age and the developmental

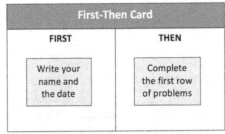

First-Then Card	
FIRST	**THEN**
Write your name and the date	Complete the first row of problems

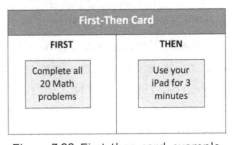

First-Then Card	
FIRST	**THEN**
Complete all 20 Math problems	Use your iPad for 3 minutes

Figure 3.22. First-then card–example.

level of the student, the activities can be visually represented using images or text. As a visual support, a first-then card:

- Gives the student a visual representation by specifying what activity (or what part of an activity) must be completed first and what activity will follow.
- Is portable, so that it can be used in various areas of the school environment. Cards can be created ahead of time using paper or a digital format or created on the spot using sticky notes, a whiteboard, or other tool to display the information visually.

Chunking Folders

To break assignments into small, clearly identifiable steps, you can provide a chunking folder to present material "one chunk at a time" to minimize distractions and help students focus on a chunk of content. These can be made from colored or manila-type file folders, with a series of flaps to cover content. Flaps are flipped over, one flap at a time, to reveal a chunk of content (see Figure 3.23). The student completes a chunk of content and then turns the flap to reveal the next chunk of content. Another chunking strategy for students who have trouble focusing or are easily overwhelmed is to simply fold a worksheet in half so that the student attends to one half of the work at a time. Chunking folders have been used effectively with students in kindergarten through high school in all subject areas (Wilkins & Burmeister, 2015). It is a simple, inexpensive strategy that works well to reduce visual distractions and lower anxiety levels when students are overwhelmed by content that they are expected to complete or master.

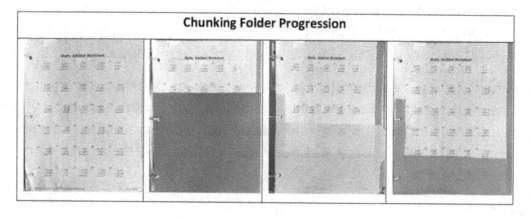

Figure 3.23. Chunking folder showing progression of work.

Highlighter Tape

Use highlighter tape to draw attention to any learning experience – spelling patterns, similes and metaphors, vocabulary words within a larger field of text; key phrases in math word problems; or specific information in a text. Highlight critical information on a worksheet, such as the directions, so that the student focuses on that "chunk" of content first, thereby gaining an understanding of what is expected before

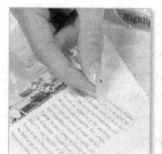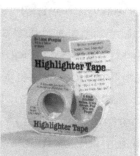

Figure 3.24. Highlighter tape.
Images used with permission:
http://www.leerproducts.com/Education_Tape.aspx.

starting work (see Figure 3.23). Assist students in chunking math assignments by having them highlight the symbol (×, ÷, +, -) in a math problem before calculating the answer.

Chunking strategies for math include grouping problems by specific operation or concept, or by providing highlighter pens and allowing students the opportunity to "chunk" a worksheet by operation prior to starting. Content can be chunked in any curricular area by highlighting important phrases, key words, or dates. Highlighter tape is easy to apply and remove, and can be reused (see Figure 3.24). It can also be written on, and comes in assorted colors and multiple sizes.

Checklists

A checklist can be an effective way to organize tasks so that a student with EF knows exactly what needs to be done, how much work is expected to be completed, and when the work is done. A checklist becomes a to-do list of the tasks that must be completed by providing a simple a check-off list for completed tasks. The checklist can be personalized to fit any task (see Figure 3.25) and becomes a memory tool that supports a wide variety of learning activities and tasks (Aspy & Grossman, 2012), including group or individual projects, homework assignments, tasks and routines at school, and household chores (McClannahan & Krantz, 2010).

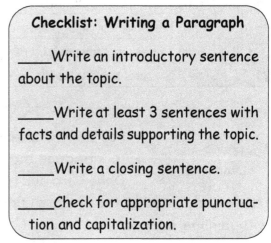

Figure 3.25. Checklist for writing a paragraph.

A checklist is a list of steps or tasks that may be printed on a piece of paper or a whiteboard, or stored electronically on a computer, tablet, phone, or other portable device. Teachers can use these to provide a list with a check-off box that can be marked with a pencil/marker, as a manipulative on a magnetic whiteboard, or electronically using an app.

 Why Is This Important?

Many students with autism become overwhelmed if a learning activity is something unfamiliar or seems too complicated. These students often lack the ability to cope, including an inability to start and to stay engaged until completion. These students need a simple process to figure out how to simplify new or complicated tasks by using strategies that work for each situation. Although there are many strategies that will support students to stay engaged, this section describes four that are universally helpful and can be used separately or in combination. To decide on the best strategy or combination of strategies, students will use *the Get it Done* strategy.

Teachers: When and How to Use *Get it Done*

Use the strategy by guiding the student through the steps of *Get it Done,* using the *Get it Done Chart* (see Figure 3.26, Appendix B). This should start as a structured lesson using familiar examples students can understand or have experienced. Move on to using actual problems as they occur in classroom or campus environments. Once students are familiar with *Get it Done,* have them put the graphic on their desk, in their binder or on their device, to be ready to use with prompts and guidance during instructional activities. In the example below, the student identifies that she is unsure how to write a paragraph. She notes options including highlighter tape, and then evaluates her use of the strategy (see Figure 3.26).

Steps	Get It Done Chart
D-Do it	I have to figure out the main idea of a paragraph. It is not clearly stated and I'm not sure what to do next or how to do it.
O-Options	• Identify key words and write them down • Use a graphic organizer, or the checklist for writing a paragraph • Use highlighter tape to highlight clues in the text that will help me to figure it out
N-Needs	Highlighter tape—I can use it directly in the textbook and can remove it when I'm done.
E-Evaluate	The strategy worked. Handwriting is hard- using the tape helped. The tape made it easier to focus on key words.

Figure 3.26. Get it done–example.

Stage 1 Learners For Stage One learners, use the *Get it Done Card* (see template in Figure 3.21) to introduce the process to the student. First, show the student the *Get it Done Card* and go over each prompt. Directly teach, reinforce, practice, and reteach each step of the process until the student can go use the steps of the *Get it Done Card* with minimal support.

Stage 2 Learners For Stage Two learners, create stories and role plays to use in which you model following the steps to solve a problem (see examples on the *Get it Done Chart*) using a "think aloud" process. Next, have students work in pairs to practice using problem situations and brainstorming answers for the *Get it Done Card*. Be ready to guide or remind the student to use *Get it Done Strategy* when you see they are being challenged by problems with getting assignments started or completed in the classroom, on campus, or in other environments.

Stage 3 Learners For Stage Three learners, as the student becomes proficient at using the process, gradually release responsibility so that the process ultimately shifts from teacher-directed to student-directed (see *Directions for Students* below).

All Learners For all learners, encourage the student to recall situations in other settings where they have had difficulty getting started on and/or completing work, and what actions have been effective in those settings. This will support generalization of this skill across activities and settings.

When and How to Use *Get it Done*

You can use the *Get it Done* process when you feel challenged by situations related to completing school work.

Use the *Get It Done Card* (see Figure 3.21) as a visual reminder: either a printed or electronic version will work. Here are a few ideas for your *Get it Done* reminder:

- Print the *Get It Done Card* on a piece of paper to keep in your reminder binder or folder in your backpack.
- Take a picture of the graphic and put in your notes app on your electronic device.
- Ask your teacher to post it as a poster in your class or near where you sit in class.

When you feel stressed about a multi-step task or long-term assignment, use the *Get It Done Strategy* by answering the questions on the card. You can write your answers or just think it through.

After you use the strategy, it's a good idea to debrief with your teacher so you both are aware of the problem and the actions that solve the problem for you.

Data Collection

Use the *Get it Done Data Collection Tool* to record student progress (see Figure 2.27, Appendix B). In the example below, class data was collected to show that students used a variety of strategies to complete their assignments (see Figure 3.27).

Get It Done Data Collection Tool				
Date	Student Name	Assignment/ Project Name	What Strategy Was Used	Assignment/ Project Completed
9/2	Jack	Book Report	Checklist	☑ yes ☐ no
10/5	Collin	Chapter Outline	Highlighter tape	☑ yes ☐ no
10/6	Allan	Math homework	First - then	☑ yes ☐ no
10/6	Reina	In-class math worksheet	Chunking	☐ yes ☑ no
				☐ yes ☐ no

Figure 3.27. Get it done classroom data collection tool–example.

CHAPTER 4

SUPPORTING MASTERY THROUGH INCREASED ENGAGEMENT

It's Mrs. Lin's first year of teaching, and she is very excited to have her own third-grade class-room. In her university training program, her professor talked about the usefulness of centers as a strategy for keeping students engaged and reducing group size for direct instruction. Mrs. Lin worked all weekend to develop centers around this week's math content, using place value to round whole numbers to the nearest hundred. Her idea was to work with one group in each 15-minute block and have groups rotate through the centers. She developed games and activities all centered around rounding numbers to the nearest hundred. She divided the students into homo-geneous groups so she could differentiate her direct instruction from the third-grade curriculum based on the needs of the individual groups. She set up four stations with the following activities:

- *Station 1 – Partner flashcard activity rounding whole numbers to 100.*
- *Station 2 – Solving problems rounding numbers to the nearest 100 on a worksheet with a partner.*
- *Station 3 – Working on a math computer game using tablets.*
- *Station 4 – Teacher-led direct instruction group.*

Five minutes into the first rotation, students at Station 1 raised their hands to let her know they were done and had finished all the flashcards. Mrs. Lin looked at her watch and realized they had ten minutes left and instructed them to go through the cards again. Students at Station 2 called out at seven minutes that they were finished, and she instructed them to ask the problems to each other again. Six minutes before the end of the rotation, she noticed the students working in Station 3 were giggling and pointing at one student's iPad. She interrupted her direct instruction to go to the group and found a student watching a video. Mrs. Lin looked at her watch and realized she had three more rotations to go. She was dismayed by the fact that students were distracted, and their behavior was getting out of control.

That night when she went home, she talked to her husband, Mr. Lin, also a first-year teacher, telling him how difficult it was to run her centers. Mr. Lin shared that he was also struggling with ways to make his instruction more interesting for the students. As a high school chemistry teacher relying primarily on lecture and chapter-reading as instructional strategies, he was finding that students didn't seem to be as excited or engaged in the learning as he would like. He told Ms. Lin that he was determined to find ways to improve his instruction so that he could share his joy of science with his students.

The next weekend, Mr. and Mrs. Lin worked together to read the research on active engagement and looked up what was best practice for their respective student populations. Mrs. Lin realized that she needed to incorporate more hands-on activities in her centers, such as file folder activities, which could be focused on prior learning. She also made posters showing what students should do if they finished their center activity early. This allowed them to continue to work independently and not interrupt other students. She also reorganized the classroom environment so she could monitor the students at the tablet center while she was teaching by putting the tablets on the table where both she and the students could easily see them. Finally, she changed her stations to increase student engagement by:

- *Station 1 – adding flashcards she had developed for previous lessons, allowing students to review their prior learning.*
- *Station 2 – replacing worksheets with hands-on file folder activities.*
- *Station 3 – developing a reminder card with expectations for tablet use.*
- *Station 4 – teaching without interruption!*

Mrs. Lin and her students were surprised to see how fast the time went by when they were actively engaged, and when she got home that night, she was excited to tell her husband about the improvements in her math instruction. Mr. Lin shared how he had incorporated choral responding and nonverbal responses using response cards to actively engage students in instruction. He also incorporated partner sharing to provide opportunities for students to process the content with their partners. Like her, he reported that the time seemed to fly when he limited his lecture to shorter, eight to ten-minute chunks, allowing students to reflect on the content and discuss what they had learned with a partner. He was amazed at how much more interested students were, and how they seemed to understand the content so much better.

Both Mr. and Mrs. Lin ended the day excited about the new teaching methods they were implementing. They looked forward to returning to their schools the next day, confident that the lessons they had planned would be interesting and engaging for their students.

This chapter will focus on the importance of designing lessons that build executive function skills, increase mastery, and strengthen student engagement. You will learn five strategies, along with steps to gradually shift responsibility for implementing the strategies to the student. These strategies will lead to greater academic success through improved engagement. Blank copies of all of the tools in this chapter are also provided in Appendix C.

 ## Link to Executive Function

Providing all students with well-designed instruction can support executive function skills through increasing student engagement, which ultimately leads to greater academic benefits and lifelong independence (see Table 4.1). Well-designed instruction is also key to reducing behavior problems caused by boredom, task avoidance, or uncertainty regarding expectations or task specifics.

Link to Executive Function			
Areas of Executive Function	**Well-designed instruction provides support by:**	**Adults who have learned these skills will be able to:**	**Real-world examples of effective EF skills:**
Developing flexibility	Engaging students with tasks that offer a clear and consistent framework, and with a variety of instructional examples embedded in the predictable instructional design.	Adapt to varied activities and expectations when situations call for flexibility.	Considers the perspectives of others in a team meeting. Understands and responds to expectations for various situations. Works on different tasks as needed.
Leveling emotions	Assisting students in achieving academic success through carefully crafted instruction designed at their instructional level, thus minimizing frustration or boredom.	Level emotions and independently utilize self-soothing strategies when frustrated.	Takes a short break when a task is difficult or challenging. Uses socially acceptable strategies to calm down, such as chewing gum, sitting on a ball chair, doodling, or coloring.
Increasing impulse control	Implementing strategies that are predictable and appropriate to students' age and skill level.	Engage in discussions, listening and talking as appropriate. Focus in a meeting (even a boring meeting) and control urge to blurt out.	Responds to corrections in a job situation. Stays focused on a task until it is completed.
Planning and organizing	Offering students instruction that is accessible and organized, as well as interesting and engaging.	Prioritize, make plans, and follow through.	Uses a graphic organizer to make connections between topics and organize thoughts and next steps.
Problem solving	Allowing students opportunities to work with each other on engaging tasks that build their social and problem-solving skills.	Recognize when there is a problem to be solved and determine possible solutions.	Responds to a challenging task by identifying any problem areas and developing solutions.

Table 4.1. Link between EF skills and increasing student engagement.

Building Learning Activities to Increase Engagement and Evidence-Based Practices

All students benefit when teachers build learning activities to increase engagement. Successful implementation of effective instruction may incorporate:

- a task analysis, the breaking down of complex behavioral skills into smaller components;
- modeling, to enable learners to develop and generalize new skills/behaviors;
- prompting, to increase generalization of target skills; and,
- visual supports to assist students in processing information (Wong et al., 2014).

These EBPs can be integrated into learning activities that involve whole-group teaching, small-group work, and individual instruction, in order to increase engagement and learning.

> **EBPs in this Chapter**
>
> - Task Analysis
> - Modeling
> - Prompting
> - Visual Supports

Implementing Effective Well-Designed Instruction: Grouping

One of the most important components of well-designed instruction is the grouping of students into effective learning teams. Decisions about which activities to teach to large groups, small groups, or individual students are crucial to every teacher's lesson planning. In this section different types of grouping strategies will be discussed, particularly in light of how these groups can support the acquisition of EF skills.

Large-Group Instruction

One of the biggest challenges of large-group instruction is keeping students engaged in the content. One way that teachers can modify their whole-group instruction to increase learning and student involvement is to offer students increased opportunities to respond (OTR). Opportunities to respond (OTR) are teacher behaviors (e.g., asking a question, making a statement, offering a gesture) that request or solicit a student response, providing students with a variety of opportunities to respond.

For students who demonstrate behavior problems, OTR has been found to increase appropriate academic engagement and correct academic responses, while decreasing inappropriate behavior (Lewis, Hudson, Richter, & Johnson, 2004). Additionally, increased rates of OTR have been associated with positive outcomes for students of all ages and ability levels (Partin et al., 2010; Simonsen et al., 2008). Common types of OTR for younger/elementary students include:

- Having students answer a question in unison (choral responding).
- Using active response methods, such as having students write answers on small white boards, hold up response cards, or use a thumbs-up or thumbs-down to indicate understanding.
- Having students explain concepts to a neighbor for a short length of time (typically less than a minute).

When designing your lessons, answer the questions on the *Teaching Style Questionnaire* (Table 4.2) to determine what type of instruction is most appropriate for your students, your objectives, and your personal teaching style.

Teaching Style Questionnaire	
Questions	**Answers (Sample)**
1. **What are my goals and objectives for the lesson?**	Students will learn about adding endings to words that end in silent "e." Students will practice adding endings to words with silent "e" at the end.
2. **Where can I incorporate opportunities to respond?**	Students can respond to questions verbally and can use a whiteboard and erasable marker for written practice.
3. **What materials will I need?**	Materials will include a small whiteboard and erasable marker for each student, along with a large whiteboard and erasable marker for demonstration.
4. **What routines or expectations will I need to teach my students?**	Students will answer together on a signal for choral responses and will use the routine for "marker up/ marker down" for work on whiteboards.
5. **How will I evaluate the level of student engagement?**	I will walk around and actively monitor participation during activities, redirecting as necessary.
6. **How will I evaluate the effectiveness of my lesson?**	I will monitor the level of participation and correct answers during choral responses and during written responses on whiteboards.

Table 4.2. Teaching style questionnaire with sample answers.

Small-Group Work

In any classroom, there may be times during the day when it is advantageous to have students work together. Having students work together in small groups can be beneficial in providing students with an opportunity to work interdependently with others and allowing them to build social skills while engaged in a shared task. In addition, small groups allow quieter students an opportunity to actively participate. However, before jumping into collaborative group work, you might want to consider the *Steps for Small Group Instruction* (see Table 4.3; Gallow, 2015).

Steps for Small Group Instruction	
Forming groups	How will you form your groups? Will you use heterogeneous groups of students with varied abilities (best for most tasks) or homogeneous groups of students with similar skills (good for tasks that will be designed to target specific skills)? It is important to form groups based on the nature of the task and the identified outcomes. In general, groups should be teacher-assigned, not student-selected.
Group task	Make sure the task given to the group is interesting, big enough for the size of the group, age-appropriate, and that the instructions are clear and easy to implement. The task needs to be something that the group can complete without a great deal of teacher interference.
Teaching students to work together effectively	Set routines and expectations for group work. These routines and expectations need to be directly taught, and students need to be given direct feedback on how they are doing with their group-work skills. Assign specific roles within the group (recorder, timer, leader, artist, etc.), to encourage more participation by all students. No matter what level of students you teach, make sure that the expectations for group participation and social behavior within the group are well-defined, monitored, and reflected upon.
Teacher's role as facilitator	Decide in advance what your role as group facilitator will be. In general, the teacher should operate as the "guide on the side," asking probing questions, redirecting, and encouraging. Instead of answering questions from a group, respond with a question of your own. Remember to be positive and develop an encouraging environment based on collaboration and respect.
Evaluation	How will group work be evaluated? Will students be given individual grades, or will the group be graded as a whole–or both? What kind of product will the group need to produce? If older students, will group members have an opportunity for self-assessment, wherein they can evaluate themselves and other members of the group for their participation in the group? All of these questions need to be considered and communicated to students in advance.

Table 4.3. Steps for small group instruction.

Group Centers or Stations

Many times, especially in primary classrooms, teachers organize students into groups and then set up stations for the groups to rotate through on a set time schedule. In content areas such as reading and math, groups tend to be homogenous. These groups of students have similar skills and are grouped together to work on a specific academic skill such as phonemic awareness, vocabulary, grouping by tens, basic fractions, etc. Heterogeneous groups are formed for other content areas such as science, where students with higher reading skills model literacy skills by reading new information to the group. Typically, the teacher works directly with one group, while other groups are expected to work independently. The general information provided in this chapter can help you develop independent work for group centers. Here are a few things you need to keep in mind:

- Make sure groups have enough work to keep them engaged for the entire rotation. Nobody wants to deal with a group that finished the work in Center 1 in five minutes, leaving 15 minutes for them to become distracted and disrupt the rest of the class.
- Assign work in centers or stations that students can do independently without a great deal of teacher support. If you group students by academic level, make sure that the independent work is truly independent for all students. If this is a concern, use activities focused on specific skills and develop routines to help groups retrieve their own individualized activities.
- Use centers as an opportunity to review prior learning. Once you have developed activities, cycle those activities through the centers to provide ongoing review of concepts that students have already mastered.
- Use a visual timer that all students can see so they know how much time is left in each rotation.
- Provide specific verbal praise for groups that are working well and following the expectations. Set up group activities so that you can actively monitor all groups without having to interrupt your teaching.

Independent Work

The ability to function independently in a classroom requires on-task engagement in an activity in the absence of adult prompting (Hume & Odom, 2007). The development of independent skills is vital to successful community inclusion and potential employment (Carnahan, Hume, Clarke, & Borders, 2009). It is a priority for all students, but it is especially crucial for students with ASD, who may have challenges functioning independently due to difficulties with the critical executive function skills of organization and sequencing (Mesibov, Shea, & Schopler, 2005), making it difficult to complete an activity from start to finish (Myles, Aspy, Mataya, & Hollis, 2018). Students need access to activities that are structured and engaging. They also need to have parameters around how to access information and materials, how to see and keep track of time, how to know what specific tasks to complete, as well as clear routines around independent work time.

Implementing Effective Well-Designed Instruction: Visual Structure

"If I can see it, I can understand it." Many students who struggle with executive functioning are more engaged in classroom activities when expectations, instructions, and tasks are provided in a visual format. In particular, students with autism have a relative strength in, and preference for, processing information visually (Mesibov & Shea, 2014). Providing information visually has been found to be highly effective, as it is accessing the student's strongest processing channel. No matter what the content is, tapping into a student's visual processing channel can support engagement and reinforce learning. Incorporating concrete visual cues into a task, routine, or activity can provide clear information about task expectations and support a student throughout the school environment (Hume, 2013).

As described in earlier chapters, visual structure can be used to organize learning environments, establish expectations around routines, make schedules meaningful, and assist in time management. Whether a student is participating in teacher-led instruction, a small-group activity, or independent work, visual structure and supports address potentially challenging behaviors in a proactive manner, increasing student interest while decreasing distractibility and anxiety.

Incorporating visual structure into learning activities can be part of a comprehensive approach to curriculum access, increasing student engagement, independence, and success. For example, using a word bank (see Figure 4.1) or word wall to present key vocabulary or frequently used words will support reading and writing activities.

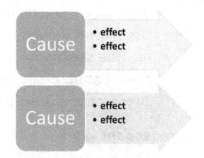

Figure 4.1. Word bank sample.

Applying visual cues helps students with autism that lack competent EF skills to focus on relevant information when working independently. It also ensures that they are actively engaged throughout the day, whether in special education or general education classrooms. Just as strengths, interests, and challenges are truly unique to each student with autism, the amount of support needed to independently complete assigned tasks varies considerably. Consistency with expectations, reinforcement, and follow-through regarding the use of visual supports on the part of all adults who support the student is essential (Sam & AFIRM Team, 2015). Ways to add visual structure to increase task engagement include:

Figure 4.2. Sample graphic organizer.

- **Graphic organizers**, such as semantic maps, Venn diagrams, outlines, and charts (see Figure 4.2), to organize content material in a visual way by providing visual and holistic representations of facts and concepts and their relationship within an organized framework (Henry & Myles, 2013).

- **Math supports,** such as enlarged graph paper to help students line up numbers for computation (see Figure 4.3); visual supports, such as cue cards for computation steps, abstract concepts, and different operations; offering manipulatives to help students grasp concepts; using drawing and/or concrete objects to help students "picture" the problem.

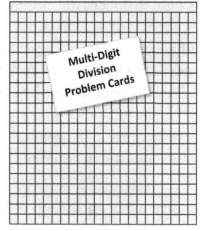

Figure 4.3. Math support–sample enlarged graph paper.

- **Reading supports** in the form of visual cues to assist students in understanding abstract concepts and comprehending new material, such as graphic organizers that help students construct meaning (see Figure 4.4). These can be useful tools in supporting students in inferring causes and effects, organizing events in a narrative, or making predictions prior to reading new material.

- **Sticky notes** to draw attention to relevant information; having some close at hand is highly recommended (see Figure 4.5). Sometimes just *writing down* what you are trying to

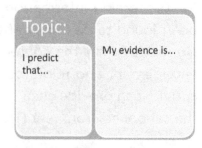

Figure 4.4. Reading support–sample: making predictions graphic organizer

communicate to the student and presenting that information to a student in the form of a note can make all the difference in his understanding of a concept or situation, and in responding or reacting appropriately.

- **Writing supports,** such as allowing students to formulate ideas using drawings, pictures, or graphic organizers/representations then adding text (Figure 4.6); providing a visual sample of the expected finished product.

- **Task boxes** are single, organized activities with a clear beginning and end. All task materials are contained within clearly defined boundaries, such as trays, boxes, or baskets, and presented in a systematic fashion with minimal distracters or irrelevant material (Henry, 2005). They may be developed for students of all grade levels and varying cognitive abilities. Task boxes can focus on academic skills in all subject areas, as well as fine motor, play, and vocational tasks (see Figure 4.7). The task boxes may be individualized to the needs of a particular student or created for use by multiple students.

- **File folder activities** are another visual support strategy that can be used to organize activities across grade levels and subjects to increase engagement, as well as to assist students in accessing curriculum content independently. Like task boxes, materials for file folder activities are contained within defined boundaries (the file folder) and may be created for students of varying ages and developmental levels, to increase student engagement by providing visual structure to tasks, routines, and activities (see Figure 4.8).

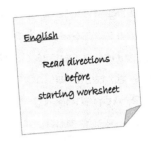

Figure 4.5. Sample sticky note.

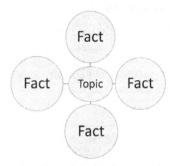

Figure 4.6. Writing support–sample graphic organizer.

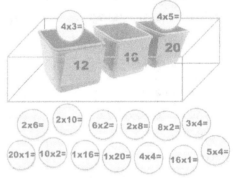

Figure 4.7. Task box–sample multiplication activity.

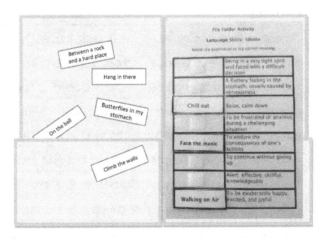

Figure 4.8. File folder activity–language skills sample.

Adding structure to classroom routines and activities can increase student engagement, leading to future success and independence. Finding ways to incorporate structure into social and academic activities requires thought and planning. Increase student engagement by providing visual structure to tasks using the *Individual/Group Plan for Visual Learning Supports* (see Figures 4.9 and 4.10, Appendix C). The examples in Figures 4.9 and 4.10 below, illustrate multiple ways in which to increase student engagement by providing visual structure to tasks, routines, and activities.

Individual Plan For Visual Learning Supports- Elementary	
Directions: Consider how you can increase engagement of your student by providing visual structure to tasks, routines, and activities. This could be in the form of minimal visual supports, or, for students needing more support, task boxes or file folder activities. Is there a way to incorporate student's interest? Use this form to record your ideas.	
Student: Louise	**Date:** 9/25/20
Type of Task	**How Can I Incorporate Elements of Structure?**
Classroom arrival routine	Provide a checklist on a small white board for student to check off as each step is completed.
Math: Solving one-step word problems using addition and subtraction to 100	Highlight words to help student determine which operation to use; provide manipulatives for computation.
Read and respond to assigned *ReadWorks* article using Chromebook	Provide a reminder card to: 1. Read the article; 2. Read and answer the comprehension questions; 3. If you are not sure of the correct answer to one of the questions, reread the passage; 4. If you are not sure what a question means, raise your hand to ask an adult.
Recess	Provide a choice board with several activities such as handball, swing, foursquare, etc. and allow the student to make a choice before going out to recess.
Social studies: Match facts with historical heroes	Structure the assignment in a task box with 4 small containers, each with the names of 4 historical heroes. Student sorts facts written on cards and matches by placing them into the correct container.
Science: Animal classification	Structure the task in a file folder with 6 photos, each of 4 different animal classifications. Student sorts photos by class, placing each in the correct matching pocket on the inside of the file folder.
Unstructured/"free" time	Provide a visual support that lists the set of activities in which student can participate during free time.

Figure 4.9. Individual plan for visual learning supports form–elementary student example.

Individual Plan For Visual Learning Supports- Secondary	
Directions: Consider how you can increase engagement of your student by providing visual structure to tasks, routines, and activities. This could be in the form of minimal visual supports, or, for students needing more support, task boxes or file folder activities. Is there a way to incorporate student's interest? Use this form to record your ideas.	

Student: _Moshe_	Date: _9/25/20_

Type of Task	How Can I Incorporate Elements of Structure?
Bell work	In addition to listing the bell work on the white board at the front of the room, write it on a sticky note and place on student's desk.
Assigned reading	Keep the student attentive and help him to maintain focus when annotating by providing highlighter tape.
Assigned writing	Provide a graphic organizer for organizing thoughts.
Language arts activity (e.g., identifying idioms)	Structure task in a file folder, so that the student who has difficulty with fine motor tasks necessary for writing can respond by simply matching idioms to their meanings.
Science report presentation	As an alternative to a written report, allow student options for presenting content, such as a presentation using PowerPoint or Prezi, a poster board, or video.
History report	Support student in selecting a topic and breaking down content into manageable pieces – research, note-taking, analysis and synthesis of information, preparing outline, writing report, presenting report, etc. Encourage student to estimate time needed to complete each component; provide a planner for student to schedule due dates on calendar.
Think-pair-share activity in foreign-language class	Use a "wait" card to remind student to wait before responding to partner after the teacher poses a question; the student uses the wait time to think of appropriate response. When wait card is removed, discussion with partner can begin.

Figure 4.10. Individual plan for visual learning supports form–secondary student example.

Flexibility: *Structured Choices Strategy*

Providing students with choices is an excellent strategy for increasing engagement and inviting students to increase their mental flexibility. Giving a student a choice can give her the sense that she has a greater amount of control, which can lead to more active participation and interest in the chosen activity (Chasnoff, 2010, p. 113).

Choice-making is a component of self-determination (Wehmeyer, Shogren, Smith, Zager, & Simpson, 2010), which is an important skill characterized by behavior that is understood to be caused by the individual, rather than by some outside force. Causal agency suggests that the student understands he is the one who can cause things to happen in his life (Wehmeyer, 2005). Students who have a sense of causal agency are more likely to act in a way that links their actions to specific outcomes (Wehmeyer, et al., 2010). This understanding can reap benefits in adult life as individuals make decisions and engage in activities that are in alignment with their desired outcomes.

When working with individuals with ASD, we must make sure that we are taking into consideration the unique differences that often affect social interaction and communication (Wehmeyer & Shogren, 2008). Many students with ASD have been taught to depend on others as they have not been provided with opportunities to be more self-directed. Incorporating structured choice-making into the classroom throughout the school day can provide students with the valuable message that they have the power to exert some control over the environment. Providing students with chances to make choices may help them to communicate their wants and needs in more appropriate ways (Shogren, Faggella-Luby, Bae, & Wehmeyer, 2004).

 Why Is This Important?

Using a choice card with two to six viable choices can increase engagement and student buy-in. Teaching students how to generate a list of possible choices and select the best option can pay dividends as students become more active learners. In a meta-analysis of research findings on choice-making, Patall, Cooper, & Robinson (2008) found that providing children with choices increased intrinsic motivation, task performance, effort, subsequent learning, and the perception of competence. Research seems to indicate that choices are most effective when students are given between three and five different choices to make, and when they are provided with three to five options to choose from.

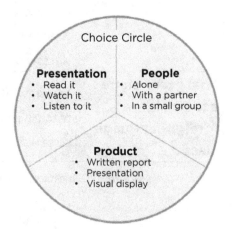

Figure 4.11. Choice circle–sample with directions for making learning choices.

Teachers: When and How to Use Structured Choices

Structured choices can be used across the curriculum to build mental flexibility and increase student buy-in. Consider the following types of choices that can be made available to the students:

- Presentation – a choice of how information is provided: through reading, auditory means (podcast, etc.), or visual means (video, etc.).
- People – a choice of people to work with: working alone, with a partner, or in a group.
- Product – a choice of how to demonstrate learning: through a written report, visual display, or presentation.

These choices are depicted on the *Choice Circle* (Figure 4.11) as a graphic that can be used to teach students how to make choices to increase their own engagement in lessons and activities. These can be used as a poster on display in the classroom and also printed on a portable card to be used as a personal reminder by students.

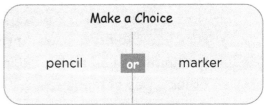

Stage 1 Learners

For Stage One learners, provide a visual choice, such as the *Make a Choice* card (see Figure 4.12, Appendix C) that provides a choice between two viable options. Start by providing choices for non-academic decisions, such as using a pencil or a marker, which story to read, a song to listen to, etc. (see Figure 4.12).

Figure 4.12. Choice card with two choices.

Stage 2 Learners

For Stage Two learners, provide a visual *Choice Circle* with three to five choice options, in three to five areas (see Figure 4.13, Appendix C). Discuss with students the importance of thinking about which choice makes the best sense, given the assigned task. Talk about how different choices may affect the finished product. As students become more adept at making choices that affect their learning, brainstorm other options for presentation, people, or product. For example, to complete a book report on *A Wrinkle in Time*, the *Choice Circle* gives specific choices (see Figure 4.13).

Choice Circle
Book Report: *A Wrinkle in Time*

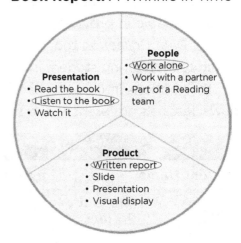

Figure 4.13. Choice circle-sample.

Stage 3 Learners

For Stage Three learners, support learners in developing a list of options for optimizing their learning. Discuss how and when they can advocate for having learning options; practice asking whether learners can choose and what choices are possible (see *Directions for Students* below).

Directions for Students

When and How to Use Structured Choices

Making choices about how you learn can be a great way to be more interested in school and to build on your personal strengths. Many teachers will provide you with choices regarding how you can learn best, whom you may want to work with, and how you can show what you've learned.

When you are given an assignment, it's OK to ask if there are choices about how you can complete the assignment. You can practice asking questions from the information on the Choice Circle.

- How information is **presented** or how you learn new information. For example, if you learn better by listening to information, you can ask for a recording or text to speech.
- How you learn best. You can ask to work alone, with a partner, or in a group of **people**.
- How you can present your **product** or what you've learned. You can ask if your work or assignments can be turned in using presentation software, or using pictures, video, or other types of media.

Remember, by asking for more choices and options, you are advocating for yourself!

 Data Collection

Collecting data on what choices a student makes in the areas of presentation, people, and product can be valuable in providing the student with information regarding his preferences. The *Choice Making: Data Collection* tool (see Figure 4.14, Appendix C) will show student progress over time, related to monitoring student independence. The data can also be used to challenge the student to try other options in order to become accustomed to other ways of learning. The example below shows Jessica's preferences and success in completing two assignments (see Figure 4.14).

Choice-Making: Data Collection					
Student Name: Jessica					
Date	**Assignment or Project**	**Presentation Choice**	**People Choice**	**Product Choice**	**Assignment Completed**
11/12	Wrinkle in Time book report	Watch movie	Alone	Written report	☑ yes ☐ no
11/15	Group science project	Have teacher explain, then read book	Small group of two	Slide show	☑ yes ☐ no
					☐ yes ☐ no
					☐ yes ☐ no
					☐ yes ☐ no

Figure 4.14. Choice-making data collection tool–example.

Leveled Emotionality: *Discussion Cognitive Script Strategy*

Cognitive scripts are typically defined as a common expectation regarding the appropriate behavior in a particular situation (Volden & Johnston, 1999). In general, people understand what behavior is expected in a certain situation, and what is unexpected. For example, most people would have a certain understanding and expectation regarding typical behavior at a doctor's office. This behavior may be similar to that which is expected at a dentist's office, but probably very different from the expected behaviors at an amusement park or a professional football game.

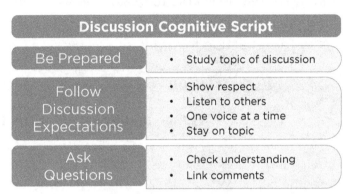

Figure 4.15. Discussion cognitive script.

Cognitive scripts are ways of thinking that help individuals to understand the expected behavior in a certain context. Learning a cognitive script for working well in a group, practicing it in a controlled environment, and then implementing it in novel environments can support students with ASD in maneuvering group-work expectations with a greater sense of ease (Wilkins & Burmeister, 2015).

 Why Is This Important?

Many classrooms, at all grade levels, require students to have discussions with others, either with a partner, or in groups. Engaging in an effective discussion requires students to come prepared, follow expectations for discussions, ask questions, and explain their own ideas (Common Core State Standards, 2018). Giving students practice with these component skills, as well as equipping them with a visual prompt such as the *Discussion Cognitive Script* (see Figure 4.15) that provides them with specific guidelines, can support learners in maintaining leveled emotions when involved in a discussion with others.

Teachers: When and How to Use the *Discussion Cognitive Scripts*

Stage 1 Learners

For Stage One learners, introduce the *Discussion Cognitive Script* (Figure 4.15) to the learner several weeks before he will be expected to demonstrate the skill. Adapt the items on the script so that they are appropriate to the age and academic level of the student. Introduce each component of the script and give examples and non-examples. Provide practice in each component and provide feedback to learner. Have student repeat each step of the script with verbal prompts until he is able to independently repeat the steps.

Stage 2 Learners

For Stage Two learners, provide practice in collaborative discussions with partners or in small groups. Collect data on student performance during the discussion. Share the data with the learner and discuss areas of strength, as well as areas for possible improvement.

Stage 3 Learners

For Stage Three learners, provide the student with practice in collecting data on his performance during a discussion. You can also support the student in practicing this skill through helping to find opportunities for him to engage in discussions with other students. Make sure that the learner knows what the discussion will be about, so that he is able to go to the discussion prepared. Prepare the student for following the script in novel situations by reviewing the script prior to the experience, and providing an opportunity for reflection following the discussion experience (see *Directions for Students* below).

Directions for Students

When and How to Use the Discussion Cognitive Script

Participating in a discussion with one or more other people can be a rewarding experience. It can help you to learn more effectively when you get to hear the views of other individuals, as well as share your own thoughts and ideas.

The *Discussion Cognitive Script* can help you by giving you some guidelines about the best way to participate in a discussion. Practice saying the steps on the script until you can say them without looking.

- Be Prepared
- Follow Discussion Expectations
- Ask Questions

After you have had a chance to practice these steps in a comfortable environment, with people you know well, try having conversations with new people in different places.

Collect data on how you did in the discussion, by answering the questions in each section of the *Personal Data Collection Sheet* (see Figure 4.17 in Appendix C). After the discussion is over, reflect on areas of strength, and areas that need more work.

 Data Collection

Collect data on how well each student meets expectations using the *Discussion Cognitive Script: Data Collection* tool (see Figure 4.16, Appendix C). The example below shows Angel's progress on two assignments after using the *Discussion Cognitive Script* process (see Figure 4.16). This data is useful for providing feedback to Angel on her areas of strength, including being prepared, and areas in which she needs to improve, such as listening and asking questions. The next step for Angel is to complete the *Personal Data Collection Sheet for Discussions* (see Figure 4.17, Appendix C). In the example below (see Figure 4.17), Angel answered the questions honestly, showing that listening and asking questions during discussions are areas she will need to improve.

	**Discussion Cognitive Script: Data Collection**

Student: _____ Angel _____

Date:	Student was prepared:	Student met Discussion Expectations:	Student Asked Questions:	Student Strengths During Discussion:	Something Student can work on—next steps:
10/2	☑ yes ☐ no	☐ yes ☑ no	☐ yes ☑ no	Being prepared for discussion about <u>A Wrinkle in Time</u>	Listening to others—mainly wanted to share own thoughts
10/12	☑ yes ☐ no	☑ yes ☐ no	☐ yes ☑ no	Discussion about recycling project—was prepared, stayed on topic and was much better at listening to others' ideas	Asking questions
	☐ yes ☐ no	☐ yes ☐ no	☐ yes ☐ no		
	☐ yes ☐ no	☐ yes ☐ no	☐ yes ☐ no		

Figure 4.16. Discussion cognitive script data collection–example.

	**Personal Data Collection Sheet for Discussions**

Student: _____ Angel _____   Date: _____ 10/2 _____

Place: _____ Classroom _____

1. **Was I prepared?**	☐ **Yes**	☑ **Mostly**	☐ **Not really**
2. **Did I follow discussion expectations?** *(Yes or No)*	yes		I was respectful
	yes		I listened to others
	no		I waited for others to finish before speaking
	yes		I stayed on topic
3. **Did I ask questions?** *(Yes or No)*	no		I asked questions to check my understanding
	no		I linked my ideas to other people's comments
4. **Things that went well:**		I practiced by talking with my parents about the book last night, so I was prepared. I also watched the movie again.
5. **Things I can work on:**		I need to practice asking questions.

Figure 4.17. Personal data collection sheet for discussions–example.

Impulse Control: *SLANT Strategy*

Students with autism are often challenged when faced with participating in group lessons, especially when new information is introduced. The pressure of this kind of situation may reduce impulse control, or the ability to stop behavior that interferes with learning. This behavior is typically related to dysregulation and can cause a range of behaviors that interfere with learning for both the student with autism and his classmates. A proactive strategy that helps students to prepare, participate, and maintain attention is SLANT, an acronym that stands for "**S**it up, **L**ean forward, **A**sk and answer questions, **N**od your head, and **T**rack the speaker."

Students who learn and practice the five behaviors of SLANT have an increased:

- Awareness of body language.
- Awareness of posture.
- Engagement in the lesson activity.
- Attention to the speaker and the information.
- Positive teacher response.

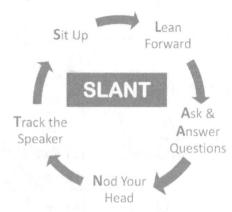

Figure 4.18. SLANT strategy.

A study at the University of Kansas found that students with mild disabilities increased their verbal and nonverbal performance during class discussions after learning the *SLANT Strategy* (Ellis, 1991). In addition, SLANT is a "Starter Strategy for Class Participation" and is included in the set of strategies related to social interaction in *The Strategic Instruction Model* (SIM) *of Learning Strategies* (2019).

 Why Is This Important?

The function of SLANT is to give the student a set of behaviors he can proactively use to increase self-regulation and attention to the lesson or activity while also increasing the teacher's approval and positive reinforcement. Utilizing SLANT regularly is a self-management tool (Sam & Affirm Team 2016b) that gives the student predictable and consistent behaviors to focus on that not only increase engagement in the lesson, but also support his self-regulation. For students with high anxiety, SLANT may also provide support as a cognitive behavioral intervention, used to increase mindfulness through early and consistent use of all five behaviors in stressful academic situations (Mussey, Dawkins, & Affirm Team, 2017). The *SLANT Strategy* is also used as a visual support (Sam & Affirm Team 2015) when the graphic (see Figure 4.18) is posted on the wall or in a portable format in the student binder. The goal of SLANT is for the student to be in control of his behavior during learning by staying self-regulated, thereby allowing him to function successfully during learning activities.

Teacher Directions: When and How to Use SLANT

Teach the strategy as a structured lesson, describing the meaning of the word "slant" by asking students to slant while sitting, i.e. leaning forward. Next, show the SLANT graphic, explaining that SLANT is also an acronym, and describe and model each letter of the acronym using the SLANT behavior descriptions. Provide a visual support by displaying the SLANT graphic as a poster, as individual printed SLANT cards, or as a picture of the graphic stored on the student's electronic device (see Figure 4.18). Next, have students practice each behavior. Reinforce student efforts and then talk about times when students should use SLANT, including:

- At the start of a lesson.
- During a discussion.
- When the teacher is giving information.
- During times when the student is feeling or acting dysregulated.

SLANT Behaviors

SLANT behaviors are effective when used during a lesson, especially when new information is delivered. It may be difficult for a student to maintain all five SLANT behaviors for the entire duration of the lesson, but encourage students to use the SLANT behaviors as much as possible. Here is a script to use when teaching the five SLANT behaviors to students individually or in a group lesson (Meier, 2013):

- **S** - Sit up: Sitting up makes you feel more awake and energetic. When you slump down in your chair, you will get less blood and oxygen to your brain, which makes you feel drowsy. It's also hard to pay attention when you're drowsy. When you sit up straight with your back against the seat, your feet flat on the floor, and your hands on the desk/table, you are telling your teacher you are ready to learn. This shows respect to everyone in the room. By sitting up, you will become an active learner and attentive listener. (Teachers, you might try using ball chairs or other supports to assist students with ASD to maintain good posture).
- **L** - Lean Forward: When you lean forward, you engage your listening skills. This will help you to understand and remember information from the lesson. You will also be in a position to write or use your hands for the activity. Leaning forward shows the teacher you are interested and paying attention to the information.
- **A** - Ask and Answer Questions: When you ask or answer questions, you are increasing your attention and understanding of the information. This tells your teacher that you are interested and engaged. Each time you ask or answer a question, you are activating your thinking and using your critical thinking skills. Each time you ask or answer a question, you are helping your teacher by letting her know what you are learning and understanding, which helps her to plan what she needs to teach next.
- **N** - Nod Your Head: When you nod your head, you are using non-verbal communication as a way to let your teacher know if you understand the information. By using this non-verbal cue, you are also learning important skills for real-world conversation, including looking at the person or making eye contact, nodding, and smiling to let them know you are actively listening. Remember to nod your head to let your teacher know you understand the lesson so that she can move on. Otherwise, she will assume you do not understand and will spend time explaining and clarifying the information.

- **T - Track the Speaker**: Tracking the speaker (teacher or student) is a visual cue that shows you are paying attention to the lesson. This will help you to stay on track and avoid day-dreaming or getting distracted. When you are tracking the person who is talking, it is easier to hear what they are saying and then to process the information. It is really important to be deliberate about this skill, because most of us have become used to looking at our phones or devices and forget to look at other people. This is also a nice way to show respect to the person who is speaking.

Stage 1 Learners For Stage One learners, introduce the SLANT steps to the student using the SLANT graphic. Show him the SLANT card and go over each definition in the acronym in order. Model each of the behaviors using direct instruction, then reinforce and guide as students demonstrate the behaviors during the instructional sequence. Have students apply the SLANT behaviors during class. Give massed reinforcement (positive reinforcer for every correct behavior) over the first week, reducing to intermittent (positive reinforcer for every two or three correct behaviors) reinforcement thereafter. Reteach as needed.

To use SLANT for self-management, develop meaningful situations for discussion and role-play that specifically address dysregulation and impulsive behaviors that have or could occur during academic lessons or activities. Talk about using SLANT to prevent dysregulation, especially during activities that are stressful or nonpreferred. Have students talk about using SLANT as a way to maintain or regain self-regulation during academic lessons. For most students, the most difficult part of the process will be identifying when they are becoming dysregulated because of stress or anxiety. It is important to guide and coach students to recognize when this does occur and to provide reminders and prompts to use the strategy.

Stage 2 Learners For Stage Two learners, create challenges in the classroom related to academic lessons and provide reminders to use SLANT proactively. Next, have students work in pairs to discuss possible situations and how they would use the SLANT card. Be ready to guide/remind the student to use the SLANT process when you see they are being challenged by an academic lesson or classroom activity.

Stage 3 Learners For Stage Three learners, as the student becomes proficient at using the SLANT process, provide positive feedback and acknowledgement. Work with the student to evaluate and self-monitor his use of SLANT and the visual graphic (see *Directions for Students* below). Have a regular check-in with the student to reflect on the results of using SLANT, using the *SLANT Student Data Chart* (see Figure 4.19, Appendix C).

All Learners For learners in all stages, encourage the student to recall how effective SLANT is in other settings on campus, such as mainstreaming, library, etc., in order to promote generalization.

Directions for Students

When and How You Can Use SLANT

SLANT can change how your teachers view you because of your behavior. When you look like you are paying attention, two things happen:

- You actually increase your attention to the task or lesson.
- Your teacher will notice and have more positive feelings about you as a student, and she will probably give you more positive attention.

You can use the SLANT process independently during academic lessons and activities. When you feel stressed or anxious because of a lesson or class activity, use the SLANT strategy by checking the graphic, doing each of the behaviors, and focusing on the activity. It is OK to SLANT for a few minutes, then take a break. When you feel your attention start to slip, it is time to SLANT.

Use the SLANT graphic as a visual reminder, either as a printed or electronic version. Here are a few ideas for your SLANT reminder:

- Print the SLANT graphic on a piece of paper to keep in your reminder binder or folder in your backpack.
- Snap a picture of the graphic and put in your "notes" app on your electronic device.
- Ask your teacher to post it as a poster in your class or near where you sit in class.

When you feel stressed or anxious because of a lesson or class activity, use the SLANT strategy by checking the graphic, doing each of the behaviors, and focusing on the activity. When you first start using SLANT, keep track of the results at the end of class each day using the *SLANT Student Data Chart*. After you are a pro, you can keep track of results every week or two. You can also debrief with your teacher so you both are aware of how you are using SLANT.

 Data Collection

Students will keep data on their use of SLANT using the *SLANT Student Data Chart* (see Figure 4.19, Appendix C). Encourage and support students as follows:

- Assist for the first few days/weeks as needed.
- Once students can take data independently, remind them when to take data, if needed.
- Check student chart regularly, giving positive reinforcement when students take data.
- Regularly debrief with students individually and in small groups, having students compare data with each other.

The following example shows the first three days Diego took data while using SLANT (see figure 4.19). By the third day, he had increased his positive perceptions related to teacher attention, learning rate, note-taking, and his interest in the material.

SLANT Student Data Chart					
Name: Diego **Directions:** ⇨ *Write the date.* ⇨ Use the key for all five statements. ⇨ In the last row, show how many times you used SLANT for 3-5 minutes in class by making a hash mark each time.				**Key:** Y = Yes N = No S = Sometimes	
Date:	1/21	1/22	1/27		
1. The teacher **looked at me more** when I used SLANT.	Y	Y	Y		
2. The teacher was **more positive** when I used SLANT.	N	S	Y		
3. I **learned more** information when I used SLANT.	N	N	Y		
4. I took **better notes** when I used SLANT.	N	S	Y		
5. The information was **more interesting** when I used SLANT.	N	N	S		
Number of times I used SLANT ⇨ *1 mark for every 3-5 minutes that I used SLANT in a 15-minute lesson.*	I	III	II		

Figure 4.19. SLANT student data chart–example.

Planning and Organizing: Strategies for Using Work Systems

Mrs. Salter has students of varying abilities in her first-grade classroom. During the reading period, students are divided into three groups and rotated through three centers. At one center, Mrs. Salter presents new learning. At another center, an instructional assistant reviews previous lessons and assists students who have difficulty with the content. At the third center, students work independently on previously mastered content.

Early in the school year, Mrs. Salter spent time teaching the students the routine for working at the independent work center. In addition, she posts a list of the activities the students are expected to complete each day during independent work time. Some of the materials needed to complete their work are easily accessible to students at the independent center; other students have to retrieve work from their desks or from other parts of the classroom.

One of the students in the class, Mia, had a difficult time getting started on the assigned tasks at the independent work center and needed frequent adult support, asking such questions as "What do I do first?," "How long will it take?," "How do I do this work?," "Am I done yet?," and "What do I do when I'm finished?" To help her student function more independently, Mrs. Salter added visual components to Mia's tasks, such as task boxes and file folders, accommodating Mia's visual strength and providing organization to the materials. Mrs. Salter also set up Mia's independent work area ahead of time so that Mia did not have to travel away from the center to access her materials.

Mia was highly motivated to go to the classroom library area when her work was completed but had difficulty initiating and completing tasks during her independent work time, so Mrs. Salter developed and implemented an individualized work system for her. The system includes information Mia needs about the process of working on tasks during her independent work time. Mia is highly motivated to use her work system as she can clearly see what work she has to do. She is motivated to finish her work because she gets to go to the library area when she has completed all activities indicated in her work system. Finally, data collected indicate that Mia rarely needs adult intervention during independent work time now, due to the implementation of a work system and additional visual structure.

Setting up tasks through individualized work systems makes learning situations more predictable for students and supports students in demonstrating positive behaviors. A work system is a presentation of tasks and materials that teaches a student how to work efficiently and independently. Work systems were developed as a component of structured teaching within the TEACCH program (Treatment and Education of Autism and Communication Handicapped Children), a comprehensive statewide program in North Carolina that serves children and adults on the autism spectrum. Work systems address individual learner needs and promote participation in classroom, home, or community settings (Carnahan, Harte, Dyke, Hume, & Borders, 2011). Work systems support students by reducing distractibility, as well as motivating them to get started and reach the "finished" point, through visually showing what tasks they are being asked to complete and how they will see that they are making progress, by answering a series of questions (Mesibov & Shea, 2014):

1. What work do I have to do?
2. How much work do I have to do?
3. How do I know when my work is finished?
4. What do I do next?

Work systems can be used with students of varying grade levels and abilities and in a variety of settings to support academic skills, play and leisure skills, grooming, domestic chores, community activities, as well as vocational skills (Wilkins & Burmeister, 2015). They provide the information about the process of working on a task or a series of tasks that supports the student in understanding what he is to do each step of the way so that he can work independently (Mesibov & Shea, 2014).

 Why Is This Important?

In order to successfully complete a series of tasks, whether it be a domestic chore, a crafting experience, or an on-the-job project, many of us use a system that visually indicates what work and how much work has to be done, how we will know when the work is finished, and what happens next. For some, this may be in the form of a checklist on a whiteboard or digital device, or through a series of photos or hand drawn icons. Some examples are using recipes, following written directions from a map, or utilizing how-to directions or online videos for household repairs. These tools are types of work systems that help many of us complete tasks and work independently.

Just as they help adults, work systems support students to work efficiently and independently by breaking tasks into small steps that create an "action plan" consisting of a set of tasks, jobs, or a routine that the student is to complete independently during a specific amount of time. Work systems help students to be more engaged in tasks and activities by making expectations clear. Implementing work systems in settings in which students are expected to work independently increases the likelihood of independent performance of skills in natural environments. (Hume & Odom, 2007).

Teacher Directions: When and How to Use a Work System

Whether students receive academic services in special education or inclusive settings, work systems can help them successfully complete a series of tasks throughout the day in any school environment. There are a number of considerations when developing work systems.

First, choose the correct format for the work system. Work systems are individually designed based on students' strengths and interests. As with visual schedules, understanding the student's visual representation level is crucial (Carnahan et al., 2011). Information in a work system is presented visually at a level that students understand, and can range from a written list for individuals with strong reading and comprehensions skills to pictures or objects for more concrete learners (Hume, 2010).

Work systems can be arranged in a number of ways, and are characterized by varying levels of representation (Carnahan et al., 2011). Work systems can include left-to-right sequencing; matching of colors, shapes, letters, and/or numbers; or a written system, as follows:

- *Left-to-right work system*: This is a work system in its simplest form, appropriate for a concrete learner with beginning-level skills (see Figure 4.20). This may also be the starting point for any learner who has difficulty completing a task independently. A left-to-right sequence of activities is set up directly to the left of the student's work area, and the student is taught to take the items/materials to be completed from the left of his work space, complete the work tasks/activities on the space in front of him, and place the completed materials to his right in a "finished" area. The work area includes visual information to let the student know the activity that he will participate in next.

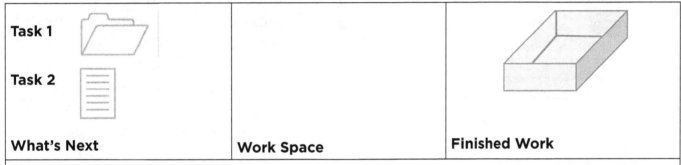

Task 1 Task 2 What's Next	Work Space	Finished Work

Directions:
- A top-to-bottom sequence of tasks is set up directly to the left of the student's work area. Tasks can be in the form of a task box, file folder activity, worksheet, or other materials. This work system illustrates that there are two tasks to complete.
- The student takes the items/ materials from the left of his workspace and completes the tasks on the space in front of him.
- The student places completed materials/tasks in a "finished" area to his right. This could be directly on the desk/table where he is working independently or in a box/container, file folder, or basket adjacent to his workspace.
- "What's Next" is indicated visually and might be what is next on the student's schedule, or it could be access to a highly preferred item or activity.

Figure 4.20. Left to right work system–sample and directions.

- *Matching work system*: With this type of work system, tasks or steps are visually represented by pictures, symbols, words, icons, or other indicators corresponding to the tasks/activities to be completed (see Figure 4.21). A matching indicator is attached in left-to-right or top-to-bottom progression. An additional matching set of indicators is created to attach to the tasks the student is to complete. In this case, the student matches the indicator to the same task and completes the task or activity represented by the indicator.

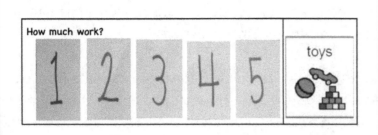

This work system shows the number of tasks to be completed as well as what the student will do upon completion. The final picture could be a picture of an activity that is reinforcing to the student (e.g., toys). It could also simply be what is next on the student's schedule of activities.

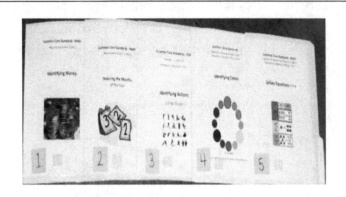

The student may start with five tasks to be completed in a 15-minute work period. Each task is represented by a picture, symbol, or number that the student removes and matches to the actual task. As he completes each task, the student pulls off the next number to find the next task. This is a concrete representation of "how much work."

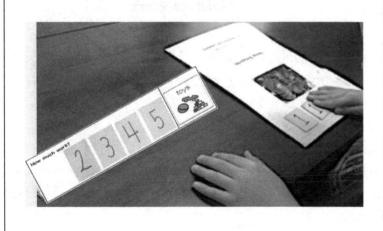

The work system consists of numbers from 1-5 and a picture of the "what's next" activity once the student completes all five tasks. After all five of the numbers have been pulled off, and all tasks are completed, the student can see that he has finished all of the work. *The Picture Communication Symbols ©1981-2015 by Mayer-Johnson LLC a Tobii Dynavox company. All Rights Reserved Worldwide. Used with permission. Boardmaker® is a trademark of Mayer-Johnson LLC.*

Figure 4.21. Matching work system–samples adapted from Wilkins and Burmeister (2015). The Picture Communication Symbols ©1981-2015 by Mayer-Johnson LLC a Tobii Dynavox company. All Rights Reserved Worldwide.
Used with permission. Boardmaker®is a trademark of Mayer-Johnson LLC.

- *Written work system*: A written system includes tasks/activities to be completed in sequential order (see Figure 4.22). For students who can match and sequence activities, yet struggle with organizational skills, written work systems are effective. Written work systems can be created using check-off systems with paper and pencil or electronic devices. The concept remains the same by giving the student explicit information about the amount of work to be done and what comes next when the work is finished.

o For students who are included in general education classes, a work system can be a list or checklist of activities or assignments for a class period that the student can check off as he completes each task. These "lists" can be developed at the beginning of the week or term and photocopied each day after specific information about assignments is written into the schedule.

o Checklists can be used in a variety of ways, and are especially helpful as a memory tool for job tasks (Aspy & Grossman, 2012; McClannahan & Krantz, 2010).

Academic Checklist: Biology Lab Project	Vocational Checklist: Morning Work Tasks
❑ Read all the instructions on the white board.	❑ Check in with head secretary.
❑ Gather materials labeled "Lab Project #10" from supply closet.	❑ Check and respond to emails.
❑ Lay all materials out on table.	❑ Check "Copy Box" for photo copies to be made.
❑ Complete Lab Project #10.	❑ Make & deliver photo copies.
❑ Place completed project on back shelf.	❑ Take 15-minute break.
❑ Place leftover materials in supply closet.	❑ Assemble 50 binders for training.
❑ Read your library book until the bell rings.	❑ Report to head secretary when finished.
	❑ Go to lunch for 30 minutes.

Figure 4.22. Written work system examples.

- *Folder work system*: For a student at any age level who can complete pencil-and-paper tasks but has difficulty organizing and keeping track of materials, a folder work system can provide support (see Figure 4.23). This is often an effective tool for assisting students in general education settings in working independently.

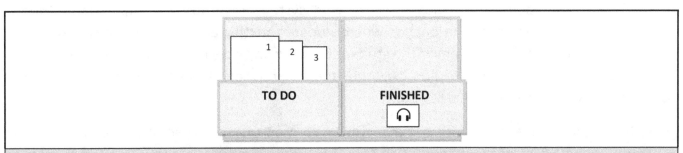

Directions: Folder work systems can be adapted to support students at any grade level. Paper-and-pencil tasks are arranged in the left-hand side of the folder. They may be numbered with sticky notes to indicate the sequence of activities. As the student completes the tasks, work is placed in the right-hand side of the folder. A visual representation to indicate what's next is included.

As students become more capable of using a folder work system, fade some of the visual supports by no longer numbering the sequence of tasks and removing the "TO DO" and "FINISHED" labels on the folder.

Figure 4.23. Folder work system–sample and directions.

Second, take into account the student's attention span on one task as a starting point. This initial work system may include only one task until the student is able to focus his attention to complete a series of tasks. To build the student's attention span for multiple tasks, add one at a time, and assign tasks that the student has already mastered, so that he will not require adult help with the tasks.

Third, determine where the work system will be used and stored. Work systems can be developed and placed in the student's work area. This may be the student's desk, at a table where other students are working, or an area of the classroom set up for the student to work alone, free of distractions. Consider movement, or the distance a student is expected to travel, when designing work systems. Are tasks within reach in the student's immediate work area, or will he need to leave his seat? Is the student expected to travel a short distance (e.g., to an area where task boxes are stored), or does he need to gather materials from various locations in the room?

Fourth, plan for successful transitions to the next activity by including a visual cue. This lets the student know what's next, as well as what to do at the end of the work time. The last activity may be something that is motivating or interesting to the student, or simply what is next on his schedule.

In addition, it is important to develop portable work systems to support students in other school environments or community settings (Hume & Reynolds, 2010). For example, having access to a portable work system in a general education setting is a significant support for a student with ASD during times when he is expected to work independently. Work systems can also be used in the home to indicate a series of tasks or chores to be done independently, as well as in vocational environments.

Stage 1 Learners For Stage One learners, set up the work system so that the materials to complete tasks indicated on the work system are in close proximity to the student, as well as the location where students are to place completed tasks. Introduce the process of using a work system to the student by modeling how it is used to complete a series of tasks. Directly teach, reinforce, practice, and reteach each step of the process until the student uses a work system with minimal support.

- Teach the work system with minimally invasive prompts so the adult and/or prompts do not become part of the work routine (e.g., prompt nonverbally by directing the student to visual cues and fade prompts as quickly as possible to maximize independence) (Wilkins & Burmeister, 2015). Ultimately, students should be able to manipulate the system independent of adult support, with the eventual goal being the ability to generalize the tasks to a variety of activities and settings (Carnahan et al., 2011).
- Teach the student where to place his completed work when finished with each task. For a concrete learner using a left-to-right work system while working on beginning level skills using tasks boxes, this may be a "finished" basket placed to the right of the student's work area (see Figure 4.20). For a student using a folder system, the completed work may go inside the right-hand side of the folder (see Figure 4.23).

Stage 2 Learners

For Stage Two learners, as the student becomes proficient in using the work system, a work system can be changed so that it is necessary for the student to travel to another part of the classroom to gather materials to complete tasks. Consider transitioning the student from a designated independent work area to his desk in the classroom, or to a table where he might compete his independent work alongside another student. Additionally, consider designating a location away from the area where the student completes his independent work so that the student has to travel to turn in completed tasks. Involve the student in developing the work system. Build independence in an elementary student by having him choose the order of the tasks in setting up the work system. A secondary student may prioritize tasks and sequence them based on length of time to complete and preference.

- As the student makes progress in using the work system, modify the work system by increasing the level of complexity (Carnahan, et. al, 2009). For example, for a student who successfully uses a matching work system and has good reading skills, consider transitioning the student to a written work system.
- As the student becomes more effective at planning and organizing, encourage the student to set up his own system in your classroom or other school environments.
- Train other teachers who support the student so that work systems can be used across settings to promote generalization.

Stage 3 Learners

For Stage Three learners, support the student in developing his own work system, offering suggestions for the best type of system, such as written work systems (see Figure 4.22) and file folder systems (see Figure 4.23). Gradually release responsibility so that the process ultimately shifts from teacher-developed work systems to student-developed (see *Directions for Students* below). Provide the student with opportunities to collect data using the *Independent Work Progress Monitoring Form* (Figure 4.25, Appendix C).

Directions for Students

When and How to Use a Work System

A work system is a visual tool that helps you to understand what tasks are to be completed during an independent work time and what to do when you are finished. You can use a work system as a strategy to help you with planning and organization so that you can work efficiently and independently.

Use the *My Personal Work System Template* (see Figure 4.24 in Appendix C) to develop your own work system. Determine if there are particular tasks that should be completed before others and put them in order on your list. Organize your materials based on that list to complete your work independently.

My Personal Work System Template	
Name: *Giovanni* Location: *my desk* Date: *Monday and Friday*	
What is the Task?	**What Materials Do I Need?**
Living/Non living sorting task	*Task box with picture/word cards*
Science flip book	*Blank flip book, crayons, pencil*
Arctic animal worksheet	*Folder, worksheet, pencil*
What Do I Do When I'm Finished?	
Go on the computer for five minutes.	

Figure 4.24. My personal work system template–example.

 Data Collection

Use the *Independent Work Progress Monitoring Form* (see Figure 4.25, Appendix C) as a data collection system to record the student's ability to use the work system to complete tasks during independent work time without adult help. In the previous example Giovanni used the *My Personal Work System Template* (Figure 4.24) to organize his tasks and list the materials he needed. His teacher used the *Independent Work Progress Monitoring Form* below to record his progress in completing tasks when given a written list work system and familiar tasks (Figure 4.25).

Independent Work Progress Monitoring Form				
Student: *Giovanni* **Work System Format:** *Written list* **Date:** *1/24*				
Place a number in the column designating the level of independence during work sessions. **Scoring Key: 2 =** Independent, **1** = Prompt needed, **0** = No Response				
	Accesses materials	**Completes task**	**Places work in finished location**	**Transitions to next activity**	**Comments**
Initial Task	2	2	2	2	*G. enjoys this task*
Next Task	1	0	1	1	*Didn't retrieve materials or start— this was a new task*
Next Task	2	2	2	2	*Some errors but completed this familiar task independently*
Next Task					
Activity when done	2	**Comments:** *Very motivated by computer time*			

Figure 4.25. Independent work progress monitoring form–example.

Problem Solving: Self-Advocacy Strategies

Amiko felt like she wanted to scream. She had been excited about the middle school history proj-ect, until the teacher announced that everyone would be working together in groups of four. She hated working in a group. Working with a partner could sometimes be ok, but working with three other people was really difficult. For one thing, it was really noisy sitting in a group with three other students. She felt like she couldn't think with all the talking. Also, two of the students in her group didn't get along, and they kept saying mean things to each other. Their faces looked mean, and they kept mumbling things to the other group members. Amiko didn't like it when people were mad at each other. It made her uncomfortable. Amiko asked her teacher if she could work alone, but her teacher just said, "No. Everyone has to work in a group."

Amiko talked to her parents about her challenges with the group work situation. They talked about her options, which included letting it go and moving on, advocating for a new solution, or letting it bother her. Amiko said she wanted to try and advocate for a new solution, so her parents worked with her to prepare what she could say to her teacher.

*The next day, Amiko arrived early at school and asked her teacher if she could talk to her for a few minutes. She told her teacher **what** she was concerned about – working in the group and feeling frustrated with the noise and the social problems of the other group members. She explained **why** it was important to her – she told her teacher that she wanted to do well on the project, but that her autism made it difficult to work with a lot of distracting noise. She discussed **what** some possible solutions might be, including working alone; staying in the group and trying to focus; or contributing to the group, but working in a quiet place during class. Finally, she shared **which** strategy she was advocating for – she was hoping she could continue to contribute to the group, but that she might have the option of working in a quiet place if the group environment became too stressful.*

Amiko's teacher thanked her for talking to her about her concerns and agreed with Amiko's solu-tion. Amiko found that knowing that she could work alone if she needed to helped her to put up with some of the frustration of being in the group. There were times that she left the group to work alone; however, there were also times when she chose to stay in the group and work with the other students. Her group finally managed to work together as a team and their finished project earned all of them a good grade.

Amiko was proud of herself for solving the problem, and for advocating for her position with her teacher. She was also proud of herself for sticking with her group, even though it was challenging.

For many students with ASD, a lack of flexibility, combined with challenges in problem solving, can make dealing with teacher expectations difficult at times, causing a lack of engagement with assignments and activities. If a student with ASD is given an assignment or activity that he is uncomfortable with, he may shut down, disengage, and stop working. In situations in which a student encounters a problem with an assignment, instead of avoiding it, he can be proactive and use a tool for analyzing the problem and choosing a solution. If he chooses to advocate for a new solution, learning a simple method for advocating for a position can make the discussion less emotional and, hopefully, more effective.

Learning how to effectively advocate for a selected solution is a valuable life skill that can be useful in school, at home, in the community, and at work. Two strategies are presented in this section. First, the four step *Problem-Solving Chart* (Figure 4.26; Mataya & Owens, 2013), gives students a process for defining the problem, and making decisions about how to handle the problem, including:

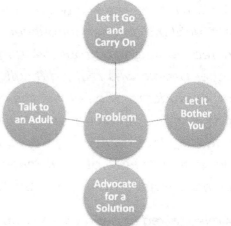

- Letting it go and moving on.
- Letting it bother you.
- Advocating for a solution.
- Talking to an adult.

Figure 4.26. Problem-solving chart (Mataya & Owens, 2013). Used with permission.

The *4W Map* (Figure 4.27) is a second strategy illustrated by Amiko. It asks important questions that will help:

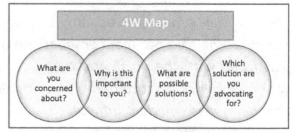

- Define the problem.
- Identify why this is an important problem.
- Determine possible solutions.
- Decide which solution makes sense.

Figure 4.27. 4W map.

Large illustrations of the graphics for the *Problem-Solving Chart* (Figure 4.26) and the *4W Map* (Figure 4.27) graphics may be found in Appendix C.

 Why this is important

Participating in learning activities and completing assignments is often a challenge for students with ASD. It is important that these students learn to be assertive about identifying and communicating when they are confused, stressed, or unsure about how to participate in an instructional activity. Once they can identify the problem, the next step is to self-advocate by identifying and following through with an effective solution that will increase their own engagement and learning success. Practicing what to say and how to say it when advocating for a solution is a valuable life skill that can be used in school, at work, and in social relationships throughout the life span. When teaching these skills, it is important to provide opportunities for students with ASD to practice self-advocacy and self-determined behavior (Wehmeyer, et al., 2010). Modeling effective self-advocacy, practicing in a safe environment, and receiving coaching following the use of the skill in other environments can provide the level of practice and reflection needed to bring the skill to mastery.

Teachers: When and How to Teach and Practice Self-Advocacy Strategies

Stage 1 Learners
For Stage One learners, discuss what options students have when they encounter a learning problem at school. Show students the *Problem-Solving Graphic* and explain how the graphic can be used to choose the best response to a problem (see Figure 4.26).

Stage 2 Learners
For Stage Two learners, have students work with partners to practice brainstorming solutions and advocating for a solution. Introduce problem-solving scenarios related to learning something new in school or on the job and have students use the *Problem-Solving Graphic* to work through possible solutions (see Figure 4.26). Introduce the *4W Map* (see Figure 4.27) and have students practice advocating for a specific solution.

Stage 3 Learners
For Stage Three learners, students practice problem solving with real-life problems and develop 4W Maps for advocating for a desired solution (see *Directions for Students* below).

Directions for Students

When and How to Use Self-Advocacy Strategies

There may be times when you are asked to work in a situation that is not the easiest for you and your learning strengths. For example, you may be asked to work in a group when you prefer to work alone or with just one other person, or you may be told you need to do an oral presentation, when you get very nervous in front of other people and would prefer to prepare a video presentation or Prezi instead. When situations like these happen, you will want to decide what is the best way to deal with the situation.

You can use the *Problem-Solving Chart* (Figure 4.26) to help you decide which solution will be the best for you. Some options are:

- Let it go and carry on – decide you'll do your best work, even if it is not your preferred way of working.
- Let it bother you – decide you'll try to do the work, even though you are bothered about the situation and may not do your best work.
- Talk to an adult – ask an adult you trust for help with the situation.
- Advocate for a solution – talk to your teacher about possible options and advocate for an option that will work for you.

If you decide to advocate for a solution, you can use the *4W Map* to prepare to discuss your idea for a new solution. If you prepare what you are going to say in advance, you will be more organized when you advocate for your solution, which can help you to stay calm.

Remember, your teacher may not agree with your solution. If that happens, use strategies that can help you to remain calm and polite. Thank your teacher for taking the time to listen to your idea and considering it. Revisit the *Problem-Solving Chart* to select another option for dealing with the problem.

Advocating for yourself does not mean that the other person will always go along with what you have suggested. However, learning to advocate for yourself is a valuable skill that you can use throughout your life.

Data Collection

Use the *Self-Advocacy Data Collection* form (see Figure 4.28, Appendix C) to record how the student uses the strategy. In the example below, Sunil's teacher documents the type of problem he encountered, whether or not he used self-advocacy skills, and whether he initiated the behavior or needed direct or indirect prompts (see Figure 4.28).

Self-Advocacy Data Collection			
Student: Sunil			
Directions: For each problem listed, describe whether the student used self-advocacy skills and, if so, whether the student initiated the use of the skills or needed a direct or indirect prompt.			
Date	**Describe the Problem**	**Used Self-Advocacy Skills: Y/N**	**Student was:** **I = independent** **P = prompted**
3/9	Was upset about the topic he was assigned for his history project	☐ yes ☑ no	☐ I ☑ P
3/12	Didn't want to work with large group for literature discussion	☑ yes ☐ no	☐ I ☑ P
3/27	Wanted to change book for book report	☑ yes ☐ no	☑ I ☐ P
		☐ yes ☐ no	☐ I ☐ P
		☐ yes ☐ no	☐ I ☐ P

Figure 4.28. Self-advocacy data collection tool–example.

CHAPTER 5

CHANGING BEHAVIOR THROUGH UNDERSTANDING THE FUNCTION OF BEHAVIOR

*T*he teachers and support providers in Shareen's fifth-grade classroom are at their wits' end in terms of dealing with her behavior. Shareen often exhibits interfering behaviors, such as refusing to participate in work tasks, disrupting the work of other students in the class, arguing with staff, and destroying property. When given a directive by staff, Shareen often loudly yells, "No!" and moves to another area of the classroom. When she is told she needs to change activities, she often throws items on the floor and yells, sometimes taking items from other students and throwing those as well.*

Implementation of a visual schedule helped address some of the problem behaviors. However, staff is still concerned, as Shareen's behavior continues to interfere with her learning and the learning of others. Data were collected to determine what was happening in the setting at the time of the target behavior to determine possible antecedents, or precursors. In addition, data were collected to determine the usual consequences of Shareen's behavior. These data were then analyzed to develop some hypotheses regarding the function of Shareen's behavior.

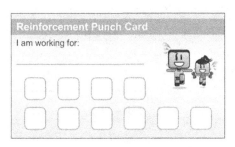

Figure 5.1. Reinforcement punch card.

School personnel, along with Shareen's parents, hypothesized that Shareen engaged in the undesirable behaviors in order to escape from nonpreferred academic tasks. The team worked to develop a plan that prompted Shareen to check her visual schedule throughout the day. They also strategically built choice into Shareen's work tasks, and rearranged her schedule so that she could engage in preferred tasks alternately with nonpreferred tasks. Everyone who worked with Shareen incorporated reinforcement into her day through use of a reinforcement punch card (see Figure 5.1) that Shareen could trade in at the end of the day for time on the iPad. Shareen was also able to take home her reward card to show her parents, who provided reinforcement at home. Data collected around the frequency and intensity of Shareen's behavior demonstrated that the strategies used by the team served to reduce her behavioral outbursts.

Helping Shareen learn strategies to control her own behavior is critical to her success as an individual in the adult world. Behavioral problems like Shareen's can challenge even the most experienced educator. Developing a theory regarding the function of the behavior and responding based on that theory is an effective means of building more positive behavior. This chapter describes behavioral theory, including the importance of understanding the function of behavior, plus specific EF strategies that can be used to support more positive behavior. The chapter provides a series of tools and examples for identifying student behavior as well as the EF strategies to support student behavior. Blank copies of all of the tools in this chapter are also provided in Appendix D.

 Link to Executive Function

Students with ASD may become students with behavior problems when the needed EF supports are insufficient or unavailable. Unfortunately, when some students fail to receive the appropriate amount or type of preventive measures to help them overcome EF challenges, inappropriate and undesirable behaviors become pervasive, and small behavior concerns become big behavior problems. Table 5.1 describes key EF skills, how these skills can be supported by changing behavior through understanding function, and how these skills impact adult life.

 Building Positive Behavior and Evidence-Based Practices

In supporting positive behavior, several EBPs are combined to provide support for students who exhibit challenging behaviors in the school environment. Specifically, teachers and other educational professionals can combine the components of functional behavior assessment, extinction, prompting, reinforcement, response interruption/redirection, visual support, and differential reinforcement of alternative, incompatible, or other behavior (Wong et al., 2014).

EBPs in this Chapter

- Functional Behavioral Assessment
- Extinction
- Prompting
- Reinforcement
- Response Interruption/Redirection
- Antecedent-Based Intervention
- Differential Reinforcement of Alternative, Incompatible or Other Behavior
- Visual Supports

Link to Executive Function			
Areas of Executive Function:	Understanding function to change behavior provides support by:	Adults who have learned these skills will be able to:	Real-world examples of effective EF skills:
Developing flexibility	Supporting students who struggle with change through predictable routines, clear expectations, and explicitly taught strategies.	Work with others and adapt to their idiosyncrasies or communicate personal needs appropriately. Adapt to changes in a workspace or schedule.	Asks a co-worker to stop tapping his pen in a meeting, instead of grabbing the pen and breaking it or throwing it across the room.
Leveling emotions	Providing students with safe outlets for dealing with emotions and providing appropriate alternatives when students are dealing with excessive emotionality.	Deal with frustrations in school, home, work, and community settings by using socially appropriate behaviors. Engage in satisfying social interactions with others in a variety of contexts.	Takes a short break to walk around and get a drink of water when irritated with a customer, instead of yelling at the customer to, "Shut up and leave."
Increasing impulse control	Providing supports through antecedent based interventions that replace impulsive behaviors with more appropriate alternatives.	Complete difficult tasks and defer reward until a task, or part of a task, is completed. Stay focused on work tasks when at work.	Rewards oneself with a preferred activity for completing part of a challenging task, instead of engaging solely in the preferred activity and ignoring the challenging task.
Planning and organizing	Offering students instruction.that is accessible and organized, as well as interesting and engaging. Supporting students to be successful with long-term assignments by teaching overt strategies for planning and organization of multipart assignments.	Finish what needs to be done by organizing time, materials, and tasks.	Has a plan for completing a difficult task, including planning ahead for breaks and rewards, instead of becoming overwhelmed and walking off the job.
Problem solving	Allowing students opportunities to work with each other on engaging tasks that build their social and problem-solving skills.	Understand what is needed in order to work productively and make changes in order to increase productivity and work satisfaction.	Makes changes to a workspace to be more functional, instead of becoming increasingly irritated, uncomfortable, and dysregulated because of a poorly designed space.

Table 5.1. Link between EF skills and behavior.

PBIS- Supporting Positive Behavior

Behavior problems, such as task refusal, disruption, property destruction, aggression, protestations, and others, can result in serious interruptions in any setting – whether in the classroom, at home, in the community, or at a work place. Positive behavior interventions and supports, or PBIS (Horner, Sugai, & Anderson, 2010), provide a structure for understanding the function of a behavior and identifying possible strategies to reduce problematic behavior while increasing positive, prosocial behaviors. PBIS is a framework that developed from the technology and principles of applied behavior analysis, or ABA (Horner & Sugai, 2015; Carr et al., 2002). Both PBIS and ABA are behavioral approaches that focus on the use of evidence-based practices to improve the quality of life of individuals of all abilities and ages (Dunlap, Carr, Horner, Zarcone, & Schwartz, 2008). Positive behavior in this context refers to skills that are likely to increase personal satisfaction and success in a variety of situations, including school, work, social, community, family, and recreation settings. When we discuss providing support, we are describing educational methods used to strengthen positive behavior and those systems designed to promote opportunities to display positive behavior (Carr et al., 2002).

A Framework for Understanding Behavior–PBIS

PBIS incorporates a three-tier model (see Figure 5.2) that stresses designing behavioral interventions according to what is needed by *all* students (Tier 1), *most* students (Tier 2), and *some* students (Tier 3). PBIS is most effectively implemented at a school-wide level, and includes the following core principles:

- Appropriate behavior can be effectively taught to all children.
- Intervention is most effective before behavior escalates.
- Service delivery should be deployed using a multitier model to provide needed strategies and resources.
- Evidence-based practices should be used as interventions.
- Student progress should be monitored.
- Data must be collected and used for decision-making.
- Assessment results are used as screening data for various purposes.

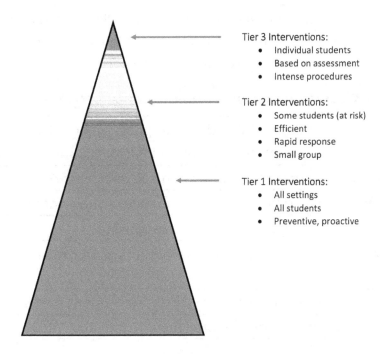

Figure 5.2. PBIS three-tier pyramid.

Tier 1 interventions are implemented at a school-wide level and are integrated into all settings with all students. The focus is to apply practices that are preventive and proactive. As such, Tier 1 practices and processes provide the foundations for strategies used at Tier 2 and 3.

Tier 2 interventions are generally provided to small groups of students who are at risk of exhibiting more serious behavior problems. Strategies used should be highly efficient, evidence-based, and data-driven.

Tier 3 interventions are focused on the individual student and based on a functional behavior assessment, or FBA (Sugai et al., 2000). Interventions at this level take into consideration the hypothesized function, or purpose, of the behavior. Problem solving around the target behavior is conducted using a team approach and focused on the individual needs of the student (Horner & Sugai, 2015). The educational team seeks to teach alternative behaviors that will meet the function of the undesirable behavior.

Setting the Stage: The Importance of Prevention.

Behavior is one of the last chapters in this book for a reason. It is easy to jump to the idea that a student has a behavior problem, prior to realizing that factors such as classroom environment, program structure, and/or learning activities may be the issue in the situation. In addition, it may not be that the student has a behavior problem, but that they are struggling to learn important executive function skills. We often spend a great deal of time trying to "fix" troublesome behavior, before putting in the time needed to fix the situation to be more supportive of positive, pro-social behavior. In fact, if you have skipped the first four chapters and are reading this chapter first, you have missed the foundational concepts regarding how to teach executive function skills that, when implemented correctly, will eliminate most behavioral problems. If you have a student who is exhibiting problem behavior, answer the questions in the *Classroom Behavior Antecedent Questionnaire* (Table 5.2) before going into further behavior analysis.

	Classroom Behavior Antecedent Questionnaire		
	Directions: For each component listed below, put a mark in the 'yes' column if it is evidenced and a mark in the 'no' column if it is not.	**Yes**	**No**
1.	Is there a clear schedule that all students can see and follow?		
2.	Does any student who could benefit from a personal visual schedule have one?		
3.	Have routines and procedures been directly taught?		
4.	Are there posters in the classroom with reminders about main routines and procedures?		
5.	Are learning activities designed to promote active student participation?		
6.	Are learning activities at the appropriate level for the students?		
7.	Are expectations clear?		
8.	Do students receive specific reinforcement for positive, prosocial behavior?		

Table 5.2. Classroom behavior antecedent questionnaire.

If you answer "no" to any of the above questions, work on structuring the learning environment to more effectively support positive behavior. If all your answers are in the affirmative, and yet one or more of your students are exhibiting problem behaviors, read on for some specific ideas for behavior supports.

To Get or to Avoid: Understanding the Function of Behavior.

When thinking about behavior, it is important to understand that behavior is a method of communication. Some students exhibit behaviors to get access to preferred activities or objects, adult or child attention, or to gain sensory input. Other students may exhibit undesirable behaviors to escape or avoid certain activities or attention from adults or other children, or to avoid negative sensory input (see Table 5.3). Understanding what the student is communicating through his behavior is key to responding appropriately to the behavior. It is also imperative to avoid inadvertently reinforcing the undesirable behavior (cf. Scott, Alter, & McQuillan, 2010).

Get	Avoid/Escape
Tangibles (activities/items)	Tangibles (activities)
Attention (adult or child)	Attention (adult or child)
Sensory need met	Sensory input (aversive)

Table 5.3. Function of behavior and components students may seek to get or avoid.

In order to gain insight into the function of a student's behavior, it is useful to analyze the behavioral A-B-Cs:

- **A**ntecedent (what occurs before the behavior)
- **B**ehavior (what is the specific behavior of concern)
- **C**onsequences (what happens after the behavior)

Collecting data about the antecedents and consequences of a specific behavior can lead to the development of a hypothesis regarding the function of the behavior (Camacho, Anderson, Moore, & Furlonger, 2014). Let's look at two examples.

Example 1:

Jared, an eight-grade student, has been getting in trouble in math class. On Monday, when students were supposed to be working on their math worksheets at their desks, Jared called the girl sitting next to him a name, and the teacher sent him to another classroom. On Tuesday, after students were assigned math questions in their textbooks, Jared sighed loudly and said, "I hate this _____ class." The teacher sent him to the office on a referral. On Wednesday, Jared scrunched his math worksheet into a ball and threw it on the floor. When the teacher told him to pick it up and get to work, he put his head down on his desk and refused to move. His teacher told him he would be sent to the office again if he didn't get to work right away. Jared muttered, "So what," under his breath. The teacher again sent him to the office, and scheduled a meeting with his parents to discuss his behavior.

A-B-C Analysis of Jared's Behavior:

ABC Behavior Data Collection tool	
Antecedent	Being given math work to complete
Behavior	Calling someone a name
	Swearing
	Scrunching up a math worksheet and refusing to work
Consequence	Sent out of class, either to another classroom or the office

Table 5.4. ABC analysis of Jared's behavior.

Hypothesis:

Get or avoid? In this case, it is helpful to look at the antecedent (being given math work) and the consequences (being sent out of class). Jared is engaging in different behaviors that lead to the same consequence – being sent from class (see Table 5.4). Our hypothesis may be that the function of Jared's behavior is avoidance of math work.

Example 2:

Aliz is driving her second-grade teacher crazy because of her silly behavior. One day when the teacher was writing an art assignment on the board, she heard the students laughing and turned around to find Aliz sitting in the trashcan. Aliz said she had tripped, then apologized and returned to her seat. Another day Aliz belched loudly during silent reading, again causing the entire class to burst into laughter. It took several minutes to get the class quiet again, and Aliz was again apologetic. When the class was lining up to go to lunch, Aliz was dancing and making faces, again making the other students laugh.

A-B-C Analysis of Aliz's Behavior:

ABC Behavior Data Collection Tool	
Antecedent	Teacher providing instructions on board
	Silent reading
	Lining up for lunch
Behavior	Sitting in trashcan
	Belching loudly
	Dancing and making faces
Consequence	Students laugh
	Aliz apologizes, and there are no further consequences

Table 5.5. ABC analysis of Aliz's behavior.

Hypothesis:

Get or avoid? In this case it is important to note that both the antecedent and the behavior vary (see Table 5.5). However, the consequence, or what happens following the behavior, is consistent. That is, each time Aliz misbehaves, she receives attention from her peers in the form of laughter. Our hypothesis in this case may be that the function of Aliz's behavior is to get attention from her peers.

If you're finding it challenging to determine the possible function of the behavior, the questionnaire on the following pages may provide some clarity (see Figure 5.3). The questionnaire is designed to be an informal way to analyze behavior in terms of function.

Quick Function-of-Behavior Questionnaire

Directions: Answer the following questions regarding a specific behavior of concern. If there are more behaviors that are problematic, choose one to focus on first, and then move on to others.

Student Name:	Jared	**Date:**	11/5
Individual Completing Questionnaire:	Teacher–special education support	**Role:**	Classroom Teacher

Part One

What is the problem behavior? (Describe the behavior as clearly as possible, so that someone not familiar with the student could understand the problem.)

Jared is acting out during math period by talking out loud, putting down others, saying he "hates this class," destroying materials, refusing to work.

How often does the behavior occur?	☐ Hourly ☑ Daily ☐ Weekly ☐ Less often
How severe is the behavior when it occurs?	☐ Very severe/dangerous (*If behavior is significant and poses a safety threat to the student or others, an FBA needs to be completed by a behavior specialist.*) ☑ Moderate/some property damage or interruption ☐ Mildly disruptive

Are there certain settings in which the behavior is *least* likely to occur?	Days/Times:	M-F / 11:30-12:15 pm; M-W-F / 1:30-2:15 pm
	Activities:	Lunch/break and PE
	People present:	Teachers, classmates

Are there certain settings in which the behavior is *most* likely to occur?	Days/Times:	M-F / 10:00-11:00
	Activities:	Math class
	People present:	Teacher, classmates

What is usually happening to the student prior to the behavior occurring (antecedent)?	Learned math concepts are reviewed with practice activity.
	New math concept introduced. In-class math work is assigned.

What usually happens to the student following the behavior occurring (consequence)?	Jared is sent out of the room, usually to the office.

Figure 5.3. Function-of-behavior questionnaire–example, page 1.

Quick Function-of-Behavior Questionnaire
Part Two

Directions: Rate each item by checking the column that describes the behavior with the following rubric:

5 = Always   4 = Frequently   3 = Sometimes   2 = Not often   1= Never

Does the problem behavior often occur when the student:	5	4	3	2	1
1. Is denied access to a preferred activity or object? (A/T)			✓		
2. Is required to participate in a specific activity? (E/T)	✓				
3. Is not receiving attention from peers or adults? (A/A)				✓	
4. Is receiving attention from adults? (E/A)			✓		
5. Does not have access to sensory stimulating activities? (A/S)				✓	
6. Is in an environment with a great deal of sensory input? (E/S)					✓

Following the problem behavior does the student:	5	4	3	2	1
7. Receive access to a preferred activity or object? (A/T)				✓	
8. Avoid having to participate in an activity? (E/T)	✓				
9. Get attention (positive/negative) from peers or adults? (A/A)		✓			
10. Avoid attention (positive/negative) from peers/adults? (E/A)				✓	
11. Gain access to sensory stimulating activities? (A/S)				✓	
12. Escape an environment with high sensory input? (E/S)				✓	

Scoring: Add up the scores for each function (e.g., A/T, A/A, A/s etc.) using the column values and write the totals below:

A/T (Access tangible object/activity) =	5	E/T (Escape activity) =	10
A/A (Access peer/adult attention) =	6	E/A (Escape peer/adult attention) =	5
A/S (Access sensory input) =	4	E/S (Escape sensory input) =	3

Analyze Function of Behavior: If two or more functions score 8 or above, choose one and develop a *Current Behavior Profile* (Table 5.9), *Desired Behavior Profile* (Table 5.10), and *Acceptable Alternative Behavior Profile* (Table 5.11). Collect baseline and intervention data using the *Behavior Data Collection Tool* (Figure 5.4).

Figure 5.3. Function-of-behavior questionnaire–example, page 2.

Once you have collected data and developed a hypothesis regarding what the function of the behavior might be, it is relatively simple to develop a statement that incorporates the A-B-Cs into a hypothesis regarding the behavior. A simple behavioral hypothesis statement typically follows this outline (see Table 5.6):

Antecedent	Behavior	Consequence
"When (student name) is (describe setting or activity in which problem behavior is most likely to occur) ...	... he (describe behavior in observable terms) ...	... resulting in (describe what happens following the behavior)."

Table 5.6. ABC analysis hypothesis statement.

Let's look at our examples from earlier in this chapter and see if we can design a hypothesis statement that describes what we think is going on. Remember Jared, who misbehaved when given math work and was then sent out of class? Let's design a hypothesis statement for Jared (Table 5.7):

Antecedent	Behavior	Consequence
"When Jared is given a math assignment to complete ...	... he engages in behaviors such as calling out in class or refusing to work ...	... resulting in his removal from class and escape from the math task."

Table 5.7. Jared's ABC analysis hypothesis statement–example.

How about Aliz, who was entertaining her classmates with her antics (Table 5.8)?

Antecedent	Behavior	Consequence
"When Aliz is not receiving peer or adult attention ...	... she engages in silly behaviors, such as sitting in the trashcan, belching, or dancing ...	... resulting in her peers laughing and paying attention to her."

Table 5.8. Aliz's ABC analysis hypothesis statement–example.

When you have gained some clarity regarding a possible function for the behavior of concern, it's time to start thinking about strategies for supporting the student in engaging in more positive behavior.

Using a Replacement Behavior: Jared.

We can begin by using the A-B-C chart from our function of behavior analysis in the previous section of this chapter to help us think about how we might be strategic in building more positive behavior for a student. Let's start by looking at Jared's A-B-C chart (see Table 5.9):

Current Behavior Profile – Jared		
Antecedent	**Behavior**	**Consequence**
"When Jared is given a math assignment to complete …	… he engages in behaviors such as calling out in class or refusing to work …	… resulting in his removal from class and escape from the math task."

Table 5.9. Jared's ABC analysis for current behavior–example.

From this chart, we can begin to outline our *desired* behavior profile for Jared (see Table 5.10):

Desired Behavior Profile – Jared		
Antecedent	**Behavior**	**Consequence**
"When Jared is given a math assignment to complete …	… he will finish his assigned work without prompting …	… resulting in him completing his work and not disturbing others."

Table 5.10. Jared's ABC analysis for desired behavior--example.

It would be great if we could move straight to the desired behavior profile; however, for most students, if their behavior has been meeting their behavioral need, it can be difficult to change that behavior quickly. It will be necessary to build intermediary steps that *teach* the student acceptable alternatives to the current behavior of concern and *reinforce* the student for using the acceptable alternatives. We will need to identify replacement behaviors that enable Jared to complete his work (Scott, T.M., Alter, P.J., McQuillan, K., 2010).

Acceptable Alternative Behavior Profile – Jared		
Antecedent	**Functionally Equivalent Behavior Strategies**	**Consequence**
"When Jared is given a math assignment to complete …	• He will be given a break card that he can use to take a 1-minute break up to three times per math class (see Chapter 5). • He will receive his math assignment in a chunking folder, allowing him to complete one section of the assignment at a time (see Chapter 4). • He will use a visual timer that indicates how long work will last (see Chapter 3). • He will receive stamps on his reinforcement card for every 5 minutes of work completed. • He will exchange his reinforcement card for a preferred item.	… resulting in him completing his work and not disturbing others."

Table 5.11. Jared's ABC analysis for functionally equivalent behavior strategies–example.

The goal is to support Jared in completing his work, while still allowing him to escape the task when he is feeling overwhelmed. By allowing Jared to take a break, and providing him with a timer and a chunking folder (see Table 5.11), we help Jared meet his need to escape the demands, if only for a little while. In addition, by building in a specific plan for providing reinforcement for Jared when he is meeting expectations, we make it more likely that he will engage in the alternative behavior we have identified.

Note: It is essential to determine whether or not the student has the skills needed to engage in the replacement behavior. If the student does not have the required skills, we need to develop a plan for teaching the skills needed. For example, if Jared does not know how to use a break card to request a break from work, we will need to teach him the steps for effectively using the break card prior to expecting him to use the card (Liaupsin & Cooper, 2017).

In addition to implementing the identified strategies, we need to pay attention to any changes that may need to be made to the environment. Are there routines that need to be highlighted on a poster? Where will Jared's reinforcement card be kept? Who will provide him with the reinforcement, and does that person require support and training in how and when to provide the reinforcement? All of these factors need to be taken into consideration in order for the plan to be effective (Liaupsin & Cooper, 2017).

When Jared is engaging in the alternative behavior consistently (as measured by data collection), we can systematically begin to reduce the number of supports needed to encourage the positive behavior. Perhaps we can start by reducing the number of "chunks" in the chunking folder or the number of breaks Jared receives during instruction. We can also stretch the amount of time between reinforcement opportunities. Once again, we will want to continue to collect data to make sure that our changes to the plan don't result in Jared returning to the original troublesome behavior. Eventually, the hope is that Jared will engage in the new behavior that we have identified in the *Desired Behavior Profile*.

Tracking behavior change.

To determine whether or not our identified strategies are actually changing student behavior, it is important to collect data on the occurrence of the behavior. The following data collection tool is not linked to any specific strategy, but this kind of general behavior data collection can help us to: (a) identify how big of a problem the behavior is, (b) whether our intervention is working, and (c) whether we are implementing the plan we developed (Pinkelman & Horner, 2017). There are three main times when we must collect data and make decisions based on the data we have collected (see Table 5.12).

Three Key Times for Tracking Behavior Data
1. Prior to developing a plan, to establish baseline information regarding the severity and prevalence of identified behavior.
2. During implementation of the planned strategies, to assess whether strategies are working to reduce behavior.
3. When strategies are being faded, to ensure the desired behavior continues to occur.

Table 5.12. Key times for collecting behavior data.

The following data-collection tools can be used to collect data on behavior easily. Figure 5.4 (see Appendix D) is designed to collect baseline and implementation data and, as such, it should be used prior to implementing the plan. Use this form to determine the frequency (how often the behavior occurs) or duration (how long the behavior lasts) of the behavior when the targeted strategy is not being used. Figure 5.4 is also designed to collect data on the frequency or duration of the behavior after the strategy has been implemented, as shown in the example below. Collecting both baseline and implementation data will help you to determine whether the strategy you have identified is actually making a difference.

Behavior Data-Collection Tool

Student Name: _____ Aliz _____
Person Collecting Data: _____ Teacher _____
Type of data being collected: _X_ Baseline _____ Intervention

Collect data for at least **three days** to determine patterns over time.

Collect *frequency* data for behaviors that happen often throughout the day but don't last for a long time. Collect *duration* data for behaviors that don't happen often but tend to last for a long time.

Target behavior (describe the specific behavior in clear terms):

Off task-attention seeking behaviors such as:
Talking loudly, making noises (i.e., belching loudly), making faces at other students, out of seat moving around (i.e., dancing, falling, sitting in trash can).

Date:	Starting Time:	Ending Time:	Frequency:	Duration:
2/15	9:00	12:00	3	
2/16	9:00	12:00	4	
2/17	9:00	12:00	2	

Frequency: number of times behavior occurred. Duration: how long behavior occurred.

Figure 5.4. Behavior data-collection tool–example.

> **IMPORTANT:**
> IF THE BEHAVIOR IS DANGEROUS TO THE STUDENT OR OTHERS, A FULL
> FUNCTIONAL BEHAVIOR ASSESSMENT MUST BE COMPLETED AND A
> BEHAVIOR SUPPORT PLAN DEVELOPED AND IMPLEMENTED.
> THE STEPS DESCRIBED IN THIS CHAPTER ARE INTENDED FOR USE ONLY
> FOR MINOR, NONDANGEROUS BEHAVIORS.

  Flexibility and Leveled Emotionality: *TABS–Take a Break Strategy*

Earlier in this chapter, you were introduced to Jared, who was exhibiting a range of behaviors that resulted in him being removed from his math work. We hypothesized that the function of his behavior was escape from an undesirable activity, which in this case was his math work. Our hope is that Jared will stop seeking to escape his math work, choosing instead to work through any difficulties, ultimately completing his math work each day. However, it may take some time to get Jared to the point where he does not feel the need to escape from math. Until then, providing structured breaks may provide the kind of support Jared needs.

Coping with the academic, social, and emotional demands of school is particularly challenging for a student who is easily stressed due to inflexibility, has difficulty tolerating mistakes, has poor coping strategies, and other characteristics associated with emotional lability (Wilkins & Burmeister, 2015). When a student is experiencing a high level of discomfort or frustration, an important coping strategy is taking a break. As an antecedent-based intervention (Wong, 2014), taking a break can help self-regulate emotional and stress levels to avoid a meltdown (Burkhartsmeyer, J., 2007) by providing access to additional materials or activities when a student feels overwhelmed or anxious (Gagnon, 2006). Used as a self-management (Wong et al., 2014) tool, students with autism can be explicitly taught how to take a break when needed, learning to independently regulate their behaviors in a variety of situations.

 Why Is This Important?

For students who are challenged by inflexibility, as well as poor coping strategies, the frustration caused by these characteristics can manifest itself in behavioral outbursts. The *Take a Break Strategy* (TABS) supports the ability of the student to take some time out from a stressful activity when experiencing a high level of anxiety. Taking a break provides the student an opportunity to use appropriate behaviors to handle a stressful situation and return to that circumstance without incident.

Teacher Directions: When and How to Use TABS

The *Take a Break* strategy can be used throughout the day in any setting. Initially, the student may be prompted by an adult to take a break before challenging behavior emerges. Ultimately, the goal is for the student to independently use the strategy in all environments when needed.

Provide structure to TABS by considering these options:

When will the strategy be used? Examples for using TABS include when the student's behavior indicates the need for a break from a problematic task, to get away from an environment (e.g., the gymnasium during P.E. because it is too noisy and crowded), or for time away from a person.

Who will initiate it? The use of TABS can be recommended by an adult or initiated by the student, as he feels it necessary to regulate his behaviors.

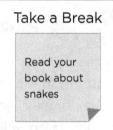

Figure 5.5.
Adult-initiated
break card with
specified activity
related to highly
focused interest.

Where will the student go? There may be a predetermined break area in your classroom, or another location on campus where the students travel to take a break, such as the office of a counselor or another adult who supports the student.

What will the student do? Purposefully specify break time activities. Whether an adult prompts the student to take a break or the student identifies the need for a break, a range of break activities can be used (Wilkins & Burmeister, 2015). Consider calming activities such as taking a series of deep breaths, using a fidget item, or drawing or coloring. For some students, engaging in a movement activity such as carrying items to another location on campus, wiping down whiteboards, or stacking chairs may be an appropriate break time activity.

break

Figure 5.6.
Adult-initiated
break card.

Consider allowing a student access to a special interest, e.g., encouraging a student with a highly focused interest in snakes to read his book about snakes or talk to someone about that subject as a break time activity (see Figure 5.5). Allow students to make choices from specified activities.

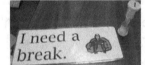

Figure 5.7. Student-initiated
break card.

How long will the break last? Set limits for how long the break will last and implement an easy-to-use tool, such as an egg timer, to monitor time.

What is the transition or reentry plan? Have a plan for how the student will know to transition back to the situation from which he took a break, e.g., when the time is up or the break activity is finished.

What visual support can be provided? Use visual supports to communicate to the student how to use TABS effectively. These can be in the form of written text or cue cards that an adult can use to prompt a student to take a break (see Figure 5.6), or a card for the student to use to initiate such a request (see Figure 5.7). Visual cues that help the student understand how to take a break in an acceptable manner can also be incorporated. This might include information regarding prescribed activities (see Figure 5.8) or activities that the student

**When You Need to
Take a Break:**

1. Set timer for 5 minutes.
2. Step away from stressful activity.
3. Engage in calming activity until timer ends.
4. Return to your work area.

Figure 5.8. Break card with
prescribed activities.

chooses (see Figure 5.9), as well as a specified number of breaks within a designated time frame (per period/day/week) that the student budgets as needed. (see Figure 5.10).

Where will visual supports be located for easy access as needed? Information regarding TABS may be posted for the entire class on posters or on the classroom whiteboard. For example, the teacher may post a list of possible break-time activities. For individual student supports, consider how the information may be accessed–reminder binder, desk, etc.

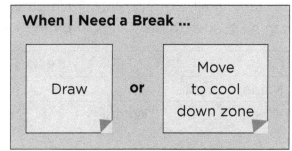

Figure 5.9. Break card with student's choices.

What additional EBPs can be used? When teaching students how to use TABS, consider incorporating video modeling to teach a student how to take a break, a social narrative to strengthen a student's understanding of the strategy, reinforcement of the desired behaviors of taking a break as it becomes habitual, and prompting to support skill acquisition, with fading of prompts as students become independent in taking a break when needed.

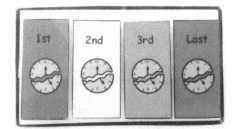

Figure 5.10. Break card for four breaks within a designated time period.

> **Stage 1 Learners**

For Stage One learners, explain that taking a break can be an effective coping strategy when faced with a situation that seems overwhelming. Introduce TABS, and explain that the idiom "keeping tabs on" means to monitor or observe something or to keep track of something. Explain that, used in this strategy, TABS stands for "**T**ake **A B**reak **S**trategy," which is a good way to "keep tabs on your behavior". Teach the student the meaning and value of the TABS strategy. Talk about using TABS to increase flexibility and leveled emotions during activities that cause anxiety and stress and provide examples for situations in which it might be effective. Have students talk about how using TABS as a way to manage behaviors will help them self-regulate when they are in a situation where they feel overwhelmed. Model how to take a break when initiated by an adult. Directly teach, reinforce, and practice how to take a break in an appropriate manner. Students should be explicitly taught how to transition to a break and how to transition back to the situation from which they took a break.

> **Stage 2 Learners**

For Stage Two learners, teach the student how to initiate taking a break. Provide the student with a signal that can be used to instigate TABS. The signal can be a word or phrase, a hand signal, or a visual (such as a break card). Support the student in determining the break activities that will best meet his needs and enable him to return to classroom work or other activities upon completion of the break. Provide the TABS worksheet (see example of completed form in Figure 5.11 and blank form in Appendix D) as a way for the student to monitor his own behavior.

> **Stage 3 Learners**

For Stage Three learners, support the student in using TABS independently in a variety of settings. Practice ways to initiate taking a break in a stressful situation. Discuss appropriate break activities that will meet the student's needs, and ways to monitor time during a break. (See *Directions for Students* below.)

For learners in all stages, to promote generalization, encourage the student to use the *Take a Break* strategy in all environments. Train other teachers who support the student so that the strategy can be used across settings to promote generalization.

Keep TABS on Your Behavior				
Name: Jared				
When	**Where**	**What**	**Duration/ Frequency**	**Reentry Plan**
Overwhelmed with math assignment in math class	Math class break area (back corner table)	Draw on notepad	5 minutes- Set personal timer / no more than 2x per period	Put drawing materials away and return to math task
Frustrated during group work in Spanish class	Outside Spanish Class in hall	Relaxation technique (deep breathing)	One-minute – use sand timer /as often as needed	Put timer away and rejoin group
Unable to cope with less structured school setting in P.E.	Walk to school office	Take walk to school office and tell the secretary the weather forecast for tomorrow	5-10 minutes / Once per period	Walk back to P.E. setting and return to activity

Figure 5.11. TABS worksheet–example.

Directions for Students

When and How to Use the *Take a Break* Strategy

Taking a break when you feel the urge to escape from an activity is a reasonable way to manage your anxiety and complete the stressful activity.

Before you find yourself in a stressful situation, think about the following things:

- How will you initiate taking a break?
- How will you monitor your time during your break?
- What will you do during the break? Plan something that is calming.
- How will you return to the activity?

When you feel like you need to take a break:

- Initiate your break, using your plan.
- Set your timer.
- Engage in your calming activity.
- When the timer goes off, return to your activity.

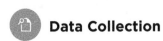 **Data Collection**

Monitor progress with the *Data Collection:* TABS form (see Figure 5.12, Appendix D) to show a student's use of the TABS Strategy. The following example shows how Aliz uses the TABS strategy, taking short breaks when she is stressed or dysregulated (see Figure 5.12).

Data Collection: TABS (*Take a Break* Strategy)				
Name: Aliz				
Date/Time	**Activity**	**Location**	**Break Initiated by**	**Duration**
2/20/8:45	Transition-ELA group	Desk to ELA Table	Staff	5 min
2/21/10:30	Independent work	Desk	Staff	10 min
2/22/9:00	ELA whole group lesson	Desk groups -3 students	Student	5 min
2/23/8:45	Transition-ELA group	Desk to ELA Table	Student	5 min

Figure 5.12. Data collection tool for TABS–example.

Impulse Control: Reinforcement Strategies

Any time we are attempting to change behavior, we must be extra diligent about making sure that we are using reinforcement effectively. Unfortunately, it is easy to get into a pattern of reinforcing the exact behavior we would like to extinguish. Let's take another look at Aliz, whom we discussed earlier.

As I'm sure you recall, Aliz was behaving in a variety of undesirable ways, in order to gain attention from her peers. What if the response of Ms. Tagaloa, Aliz's teacher, was to write Aliz's name on the board each

> Reinforcement is generally understood to be any behavioral consequence that increases the occurrence of a behavior.

time she misbehaved? What if Ms. Tagaloa stopped her lesson every time Aliz belched loudly, talking to Aliz directly (in front of the class) about manners? Can you see how Ms. Tagaloa's responses to Aliz's misbehavior might actually misfire, by providing Aliz with even more attention whenever she misbehaves? In the case of a student who is motivated by attention seeking, it is imperative that we switch things around so that the student learns how to get attention through behaving appropriately, not misbehaving.

This is the problem with behavioral techniques that instruct teachers to put students' names on the board and add check marks for misbehavior. If the behavior is rooted in attention seeking, making note of it can have the opposite effect. So, what to do?

 Why Is This Important?

Remembering to praise students, especially students who often engage in difficult behaviors, can be challenging. However, it's a worthwhile endeavor. In fact, research has been showing the effectiveness of teachers' use of specific, sincere, contingent, child-focused praise for close to 50 years (Floress, Beschta, Meyer, & Reinke, 2017). Areas in which the skillful use of praise has shown positive results include academic responding (Sutherland, Copeland, & Wehby, 2001a), work completion and accuracy (Alber, Heward, & Hippler, 1999; Craft, Alber, & Heward, 1998), following directions (Goetz, Holmberg, & LeBlanch, 1975; Hall et al., 1971), and an increase in engagement and on-task behavior (Partin et al., 2010; Broden, Bruce, Mitchell, Carter, & Hall, 1970; Ferguson & Houghton, 1992; Sutherland, Wehby, & Copeland, 2000).

Teacher Directions: When and How to Use Reinforcement

Three kinds of praise are generally used in classrooms to reinforce student behavior (Marchant & Anderson, 2012): general, effective, and instructive. Table 5.13 outlines these three types and the effect they have on student behavior, and gives an example of each type.

Type of Praise	Example	Effect on Behavior
General praise	"Good job!" in response to a student putting away materials at the end of a lesson.	General praise has been shown to have little effect on students in the classroom.
Effective praise (also known as "specific praise")	"Good job putting your materials away without being asked. I appreciate it!"	Effective praise has a greater effect on student behavior because it links the praise with the specific action that is being praised.
Instructive praise	"Good job putting your materials away without being asked. Now the class can go onto our next activity without any wasted time."	Instructive praise is most effective because it links the praise and the specific action being praised, with the rationale or natural consequence.

Table 5.13. Types of praise and their effect on behavior.

All Learners

Reinforcement is effective for all students at all stages, but imperative for students who are at risk for behavioral challenges. Unfortunately, it is these types of students who generally receive the least amount of positive reinforcement and the greatest amount of corrective feedback in classrooms (Partin et al., 2010). In addition, these at-risk students receive more teacher attention in response to their inappropriate behavior and less teacher attention for engaging in appropriate behavior (Partin et al., 2010).

Admittedly, it can be difficult to remember to reinforce the appropriate behavior of a student who misbehaves often. Many times, the teacher simply feels a sense of relief that the student is not misbehaving and doesn't want to interrupt the appropriate behavior for fear of setting off another bout of misbehavior. This is understandable; however, it is extremely important to *remember to provide students with reinforcement for the behaviors we are attempting to increase.*

Data Collection

One of the most effective ways to increase the use of reinforcing statements in classrooms is teacher self-monitoring (Partin et al., 2010; Pinkelman & Horner, 2017). The easiest way to do this is to record a 15-minute segment of a lesson, then choose a five minute sample and tally each time you praise either a student or a group of students. Figure 5.13 is an example showing the number of times the teacher provided praise statements and corrective statements, and the ratio between positive and negative. The goal should be to make at least four positive praise statements for every negative or corrective statement (Marchant & Anderson, 2012).

		Teacher Self-Monitoring of Positive to Negative Statements			
Teacher Name: _Ms. Tagaloa_			**Data collected by:** _Ms. Alvarez, Beh. Support_		
Directions: Count the number of times you make positive statements (statements praising a student or group of students) and negative statements (ones that are corrective).					
Date	**Time**	**Lesson/Activity**	**# Positive**	**# Negative**	**Ratio of positive/ negative**
2/20	8:45-9:00	Transition to ELA Groups & Lesson Intro	⫽⫻ /	⫽⫻ ////	6 to 9
2/21	10:30-10:45	Independent work	⫽⫻ ////	⫽⫻	9 to 5
2/22	9:00-9:15	ELA whole group lesson-Review	⫽⫻ ⫽⫻ //	⫽⫻	12 to 5
2/23	8:45-9:00	Transition to ELA Groups & Lesson Intro	⫽⫻ ⫽⫻	⫽⫻ ///	10 to 8

Figure 5.13. Data-collection tool for positive vs. negative feedback ratio–example.

Figure 5.13 may also be used by administrators or instructional coaches to provide data for teachers regarding their use of positive and negative statements. For even greater effectiveness, the number of positive statements made in five minutes can be multiplied by three, giving a number of positive statements in 15 minutes. This number can then be charted on a line graph, and the teacher can monitor improvement over time. Don't forget to set personal goals and then reward yourself when you reach them.

Planning & Organization and Problem Solving: *I'm OK Strategy*

*RJ, a student with ASD, was preparing to transition to high school as a ninth grader. After a successful eighth-grade year of receiving all services in the general education classroom, RJ was determined to continue with his success in high school. RJ talked to his eighth-grade educational specialist, Mr. Hernandez, who had supported RJ's transition to all general education classes during middle school. Knowing that sensory challenges were likely to be an area of concern, RJ and Mr. Hernandez identified what might be some potential problems. In the past, RJ had experienced problems in the general education class when the sensory input (e.g., noise, crowded areas, sudden changes in activity level of the class) became too overwhelming, resulting in RJ running out of the classroom. RJ knew he would need to have some strategies in place in order to support him in dealing with the sensory challenges he might experience. Mr. Hernandez suggested that they might use the "I'm OK Strategy" to develop a plan. The "I'm OK Strategy" is a precorrection that supports teachers and students in **I-identifying** potential problems, M-**making** a plan, O-**organizing** the needed supports, and K-**keeping cool** through knowing potential triggers and responding appropriately.*

In order to know more about what challenges RJ might experience at the high school, Mr. Hernandez contacted the educational specialist at the high school and scheduled an appointment to visit the high school in the summer, before the start of school. RJ and Mr. Hernandez used an environmental checklist to analyze the classrooms to which RJ was assigned. They then made a plan for specific strategies that RJ might use to help him with his sensory needs.

Prior to the first day of school, RJ and his parents organized the things he would need in order for him to keep his cool in his high school classes. The environmental checklist had identified that noise might be a problem, so RJ included noise-reduction headphones in his backpack. RJ also knew that having a fidget handy was a good idea for a strategy to help him deal with his sensory needs. Finally, Mr. Hernandez worked with RJ's new teachers to implement the "Take a Break Strategy" that had supported RJ when he first transitioned into all general education classes. The "Take a Break Strategy" allowed RJ to request a one-minute break up to three times in a one-hour class. RJ rarely used all three breaks, but was comforted by the idea that he could take the breaks if he needed to.

For many students with autism, sensory processing difficulties may interfere with basic life functions. Some students with ASD may demonstrate a hypersensitivity to sensory experiences, whereas others may exhibit a hyposensitivity, or lower level of responsiveness. Individuals with ASD may experience challenges in any of the sensory systems: touch, smell, sight, taste, or hearing. In addition, the vestibular system, which is the system that provides information to our brain regarding where our body is in space and where we are moving and at what speed, may be affected. Another system that may be impacted is the proprioceptive system, which lets our brains know our position in space, as well as a general awareness of the body, leading to coordinated movement (Rogers & Short, 2010).

Precorrection is an antecedent-based instructional strategy that is designed to reduce the likelihood of a predictable problem behavior occurring and increase the probability that more positive pro-social behavior will transpire (Ennis, Royer, Lane, & Griffith, 2017). Precorrection is a versatile strategy that can be utilized with students of all grade levels, and in a variety of settings. It is also a strategy that can be explicitly taught, so that students can independently identify and implement precorrections that work for them. Using a precorrection strategy to identify possible sensory challenges and plan for appropriate ways to deal with such challenges can provide support for students in a variety of settings.

Precorrection can also be used as a priming strategy when it is used by teachers to remind students of expectations. Teachers might precorrect a group of students by reminding students of the expected behavior during the following activities:

- Prior to an assembly: "Remember, students, we are going to walk in a line to the gymnasium, voice levels at zero. We are going to sit quietly in our seats and listen to the people speaking at the assembly. After the assembly we will return to our classroom quietly and by walking in a line."
- Before going to the library: "Remember that we will treat the books in the library with respect, we will use quiet voices, and we will walk to and from the library."

 Why Is This Important?

Our senses provide valuable information regarding the world around us; however, when an individual experiences sensory processing difficulties that result in dysregulation, unexpected behaviors may follow. Individuals who experience emotional dysregulation related to sensory processing challenges may benefit from precorrection strategies that can provide sensory support prior to a behavioral incident occurring.

Teacher Directions: Planning and Problem Solving for *I'm OK Strategy*

Stage 1 Learners

For Stage One learners, use the *Classroom Environment Checklist* (see Figure 2.15, Chapter 2) to identify potential problem areas in the classroom and develop a *Student Environmental Preference Checklist* (Figure 2.16, Chapter 2) to detail student preferences. Make a plan for possible precorrections for problem behaviors linked to sensory dysregulation. Organize the supports needed for the student to maintain regulation and have those supports easily accessible. Know potential triggers that may result in behavioral challenges and actively prompt the student to use needed support before dysregulation becomes overwhelming.

Stage 2 Learners

For Stage Two learners, introduce the *I'm OK* model and discuss the idea of sensory processing difficulties. Talk about the importance of having a plan in place prior to experiencing the need to escape or react in an unexpected way. Have students discuss how they feel when their sensory needs are not being met, and how they can identify when they need support to maintain their equilibrium. Introduce the PLACE strategy (see Figure 2.19, Chapter 2) as a tool for identifying what supports might be needed. Finally, monitor the student for signs of dysregulation and prompt him to utilize identified supports.

| Stage 3 Learners | For Stage Three learners, provide coaching and support as the student uses the *I'm OK* process (see Figure 5.14) independently and in a variety of locations. Gradually release responsibility as the student demonstrates an ability to use |

the process as a way to identify and utilize needed supports (See *Directions for Students* below).

I'm OK Precorrection Strategy			
I'	**M**	**O**	**K**
Identify potential problems	**M**ake a plan	**O**rganize supports	**K**now the triggers and keep cool
Do an environmental analysis using the *Classroom Environment Checklist* (Chapter 2). Identify areas that could prove problematic.	Make a plan in advance for how you might deal with different problems. Use the PLACE strategy (Chapter 2) to identify possible solutions.	Organize the supports needed to function well in the environment. If taking a break is a viable strategy, make sure a *Take a Break* card is available (Chapter 5). If headphones, a fidget, or other sensory item is needed, make sure they are available.	Know potential triggers and pay attention to indicators of dysregulation occurring. Make a change before the sensory issues become overwhelming. Use the SOS strategy (Chapter 2) to self-regulate.

Figure 5.14. I'm OK precorrection strategy.

Directions for Students

When and How to Use I'm OK

You can use *I'm OK* to identify potential sensory problems that may occur in an environment. Once you have identified potential problems, make a plan for how you can provide the supports you will need to deal with sensory issues.

1. Organize the supports you will need *before* you are in the situation.
2. Know your triggers and monitor yourself so that you can keep cool.
3. If you start feeling a sense of dysregulation, use the *SOS Strategy* (*Step Out and Self-Regulate*) from Chapter Two or use a *Take a Break* card (see Figure 5.7) to take a one-minute break.
4. You can also choose to use headphones, a fidget, or any other sensory support that works for you.
5. Make sure that you pay attention to how you are feeling and use your supports before it is too late.

 Data Collection

Use the *Precorrection Data Collection* system (see Figure 5.15, Appendix D) to record how the student uses the *I'm OK* strategy by documenting the setting that has been identified by the student as potentially problematic and the specific problems that occur. Describe the supports that the student has chosen in advance. Following an instance in which the student has participated in the identified situation, document which supports were used and whether the student initiated use of those supports. Ask the student to reflect on the situation and whether or not he found the use of the supports positive, negative, or neutral. The example shown below shows the strategies RJ used and his feedback about how the strategies worked (see Figure 5.15).

Precorrection Data Collection							
Student name: RJ							
Setting: Participation in group activities in the classroom and on campus							
Potential problems: Noise, sudden change, closeness and movement of others in the classroom							
Supports identified: Headphones, fidgets, breaks							
Date	**Supports Used**	**Independently Used Supports**			**Student Feedback**		
		Yes	**No**	**Partial**	**Positive**	**Negative**	**Neutral**
3/2	Headphones-Break Card	X			X		
3/5	Headphones- fidget			X			X
3/6	Headphones-Break Card	X			X		

Figure 5.15. Precorrection data collection–example.

CHAPTER 6
DEVELOPING SKILLS FOR FUTURE INDEPENDENCE

Angelica is a high school senior and is in the work-study program, attending classes in the morning, and working at Pet Depot, a local dog grooming and training center, each afternoon. She wants to have a career working with animals and has considered dog trainer, pet groomer, and veterinary assistant. In her work-study career course, Angelica researched each career and learned that she would need to improve her math and science grades to be accepted into any of these training programs. At her transition IEP meeting, Angelica's math teacher said she needed to bring her grade up by getting her homework assignments turned in on time. During the meeting, Angelica's mom told the IEP team that she and Angelica just worked on making a visual schedule on her phone with alarms set for the things she did every day, including homework, workout, and preparing for bed. She had used a visual schedule during elementary and middle school and realized she would probably always need to use a schedule to stay on track. The IEP team added a transition goal to support her by providing weekly math tutoring and daily assignment reminders. Her other transition goals were focused on building her Career Search Portfolio and Networking list to prepare for job searching.

Angelica was happy at her work-study placement until her supervisor, Ms. Ryan, told her that, although she was great with the animals, she needed to improve her communication skills. Recently, Angelica had a tough day because her bus was late picking her up for work, she forgot her ID tag, and couldn't clock-in for her shift. It seemed like things had smoothed out for the day until Ms. Ryan called her into the office and said, "Angelica, a customer complained that you were rude when she asked for help finding the dog food. You know where the dog food is stocked. Why did you ignore her and walk away?" Angelica shared that she'd had a hard day and was stressed because of the bus and ID tag, and became more anxious when the customer poked her arm and talked in a loud voice. She told Ms. Ryan that after the customer touched her, she used her 5-Point Scale and realized she was at a 4, so she walked away to avoid a negative reaction, like yelling or even throwing something. Ms. Ryan told her she was really happy that she used her 5-Point Scale and glad that it worked to help her calm down. She and Angelica had talked about using the 5-Point Scale earlier when she'd had a stressful day. She also told Angelica that they would practice ways to handle difficult customers, including thinking of appropriate things to say, such as, "Let me get help for you."

This chapter will focus on the importance of teaching powerful strategies that give students the tools to master executive function skills leading to success in adult life. You will learn five powerful strategies, along with steps students can use to become fully independent in effectively handling situations as they transition from school to adult life. Blank copies of all of the tools in this chapter are also provided in Appendix E.

Skills Needed for Future Independence

Most high school graduates are excited and ready for their next steps into adulthood. They eagerly look forward to new experiences and embrace the changes that come with their next steps, such as entering college or starting a new job. These graduates look forward to the unknown and are confident they can successfully meet new people, explore new places, and experience different activities. They have learned strategies and skills to enhance their natural ability to understand and navigate unfamiliar environments and social situations.

But unlike most of her typical peers, Angelica did not naturally understand the social conventions and rules for surviving high school, socially or academically. Angelica's autism required accommodations and strategies for every environment, activity, and social situation, to allow her to safely and successfully navigate daily challenges, both big and small. In fact, she needed to learn strategies for planned and familiar activities, as well as unexpected events.

According to data from the National Longitudinal Transition Study-2 (Shogren & Plotner, 2012), Angelica belongs to the group of students who face the greatest hurdles for successful transition from high school to a productive adult life, as Angelica and her peers with autism have the lowest rate of paid employment of students with disabilities. In addition, 36% of young adults with autism are not engaged in education or employment for two years after high school, leaving most of them sitting at home day after day (Roux et al., 2015).

Falling Off a Cliff

While in school, most students with disabilities have an IEP that provides specialized services to support post-school success. Federal law mandates these services, and they can become a safety net for some families. However, once students complete school, that safety net is gone, and there is no federal mandate for adult services. In addition, the adult services that are available have different eligibility rules and application processes, and can be challenging to navigate. Young adults with ASD may find they are not eligible for the same level of services as they received in school. According to the *National Autism Indicators Report: Transition into Young Adulthood* (Roux et al., 2015), each year 50,000 students with ASD leave school, creating an urgent need for adult services and support for this group of young adults with very unique strengths, abilities, and challenges. Unfortunately, the families of these young adults are faced with a lack of services when they need it the most, causing them to feel as if they have fallen off a cliff.

Link to Executive Function

Many of the challenges for this group are related to poor executive function skills, affecting how the young adult perceives situations, sequences steps to complete a task, focuses and attends to tasks and activities, and organizes and prioritizes his belongings, work spaces and time (Perry, 2009). Areas that most affect successful transition to adult activities are shown in the table below. These skills are foundational to success at home, at school, in the community, and on the job. In fact, executive function skill deficits often cause young adults to get fired from their jobs. Schools have an obligation to provide training and support guided by educational and transition goals that will give these students opportunities to learn, practice, and apply these skills, as shown in Table 6.1. Each chapter of this book gives teachers and students strategies to increase executive function skills needed for success throughout school and into a career.

Link to EF Skills			
Areas of Executive Function	**A well-planned transition from school to career provides support by:**	**Adults who have learned these skills will be able to:**	**Real-world examples of effective EF skills:**
Developing Flexibility	Making and using schedules with planned changes and adjustments. Defining established routines in order to make deliberate changes, working through the changes, and then debriefing after each situation.	Adapt to changes at school, home, work, and community by making adjustments and moving on to the next activity.	Adjusts tasks at work when asked to do a different job. Reschedules when an appointment is cancelled.
Leveling Emotions	Reducing frustration and anxiety by determining triggers and then putting preventive supports in place to monitor and reduce emotional responses and prevent dysregulation.	Understand causes of frustration and anxiety and use strategies, such as timers and alarms to stay on task at work, and conversation starters in social situations.	Decreases stress when tasks change at work by using a "change" signal on a personal visual schedule.
Increasing Impulse Control	Learning coping strategies that support self-regulation, such as monitoring heart rate and taking breaks when it becomes elevated, practicing regular deep breathing, and avoiding situations and people that cause uncontrolled emotional reactions.	Control self-regulation by monitoring stress and anxiety, then take action by using calming strategies to reduce impulsive reactions.	Keeps track of stressful events at home and work and uses calming app before becoming impulsive.

Planning and organizing	Understanding and using visual organizational tools to effectively manage time and assignments at school and work.	Increase productivity and control stress by using strategies that help with structuring the steps for planning and organizing daily tasks.	Uses a step-by-step structured networking strategy for organizing a job search.
Problem Solving	Knowing when there is a problem, and how to generate and evaluate solutions . Predicting typical problems that may occur in daily situations and practicing how to solve them by finding multiple solutions through role-play, discussion, and practice with debriefing after each situation.	Identify a problem by recognizing signals, such as reactions from other people, and then take action to try solutions until the problem is solved.	Recognizes when there is a problem and calmly works through a process to find a solution. Gets help to solve a problem when it seems like the issue will not go away.

Table 6.1. Link between EF skills and future independence in adult life.

 Building Future Skills and Evidence–Based Practices

IDEA mandates that schools provide transition services to prepare students with disabilities for adult life. However, research indicates that many of these students, especially those with autism and related disabilities, struggle with post-school outcomes, including college/training, employment, and independent living (Newman et al., 2011). In fact, young adults with autism and related disabilities have far greater challenges than their peers in most post-school outcomes, with employment as the most important indicator of a successful adult life (Gerhardt, 2017).

Evidence-based practices and predictors in secondary transition have been identified by the National Technical Assistance Center on Transition (NTACT, 2015; Test, Fowler, & Kohler, 2016). Currently, there are 11 EBPs, 47 research-based practices, and 73 promising practices (Test et al., 2016) organized around education, employment, and independent living. In addition, the NTACT has identified 20 evidence-based predictors of post-school employment, education, and independent living success (See Appendix E: Chapter 6). These are also organized within the three areas of education, employment and independent living (Test et al., 2016). Executive function deficits affect each of these areas, increasing the need to combine EF strategies with transition EBPs.

Transition skills taught in school rely on evidence-based practices to increase student success, including: task analysis to break complex tasks into a sequence of smaller tasks, allowing the student to learn and practice each step; self-management skills at school and in job training through use of organizational tools, such as calendars, schedules, timers, check-off lists, and other visual and auditory supports using low and high tech materials and devices (Riffel et al., 2005; Wong et al., 2014); visual prompts that act as an antecedent-based intervention by providing a visual cue to prevent a potential negative behavior from occurring (Sam et al., 2016a).

Developing Strategies for Future Independence

Successfully transitioning from high school to adult life requires years of preparation. Being smart is not enough! As students go through high school, focusing only on academics may limit their success with transitioning into next steps such as college, training, or a job. Along with academics, students with EF deficits need explicit instruction in the areas shown in the *Link to EF Skills* chart (Table 6.1) to increase executive function skills (Freedman, 2010). These EF skill areas are critical to future success, as described below:

- **Flexibility.** *"Change is a choice!"* Many young adults with ASD and related disabilities seem to "get stuck" due to their need for consistent routines and difficulty making transitions. They may also persist in talking about their "area of interest," making conversations one-sided and, therefore, off-putting to others. When faced with a problem, they may keep trying the same solution, even if it does not work.

  Young adults can work on building flexibility by trying new things that challenge their thinking, such as deliberately changing daily routines, meeting and learning about new people, going to different places for new experiences, and playing games that require strategy (Whitney, 2017).

- **Leveling emotions.** *"I know myself."* Self-awareness leads to greater understanding of their disability for young adults, and is especially critical for those with EF deficits. Self-awareness allows them to identify their strengths and weaknesses and, most important, their self-regulation states, both physical (hungry, cold, sensory, etc.) and emotional (happy, sad, angry, etc.). Specific strategies and supports for recognizing and managing stress and anxiety will increase self-regulation.

  Young adults can take a proactive approach to increasing emotional and physical self-regulation by participating in activities such as sports, fitness/workouts, yoga, meditation, playing a musical instrument, playing strategy board games, solving logic puzzles, and playing computer games that require monitoring and fast reactions (Center on the Developing Child, 2014).

- **Impulse control.** *"Think before you act!"* This is a concept to live by for most young adults, and especially those with ASD and EF deficits, who otherwise run the risk of interrupting, disrupting, ignoring personal space, and compromising their own safety. Some young adults with ASD easily become dysregulated when they experience high anxiety, resulting in negative behavior. A proactive approach for young adults who lack impulse control is to increase healthy habits by scheduling downtime, getting enough sleep, eating healthy food, and adhering to regular exercise routines (Dipedeo, Storlie, & Johnson, 2015).

- **Planning and organization**. *"One step at a time."* Many young adults with ASD and EF deficits struggle with planning to develop goals, and the steps and time needed to achieve those goals. They also often fail to organize and develop systems to keep track of work assignments. Many have difficulty keeping their personal belongings organized, allowing them to find the things they need to get their work done.

  For planning, young adults with ASD can improve their skills by completing activities, such as mazes, naming or diagramming the steps for a task such as making a sandwich, or filling out an application form (Freedman, 2010). They may find they can track events more successfully by prioritizing tasks and setting deadlines using to-do lists, calendar/schedule planners, hanging white boards, or electronic planners and software apps on a tablet, computer, and/or smartphone.

- **Problem solving**. *"Do I need help?"* Young adults with ASD and EF deficits often cannot identify when they have a problem, and may be resistant to asking for help once they realize they have a problem. They may also focus on just one aspect of the problem or be unable to identify the most relevant part of the problem.

  To increase their ability to recognize and solve problems, young adults with ASD may experience success using a checklist of tasks to be completed at home or on the job. In addition, they may use a list that breaks a task down into discrete steps (e.g., task analysis for the morning grooming routine).

The following strategies should be introduced in elementary school with modeling, support and practice. As students practice these strategies through elementary and middle school, they will have opportunities to increase their level of independence during high school to be ready for their transition to adult life.

Flexibility: *PLAN Strategy*

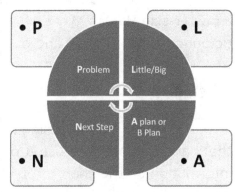

Angelica's work-study training position was scheduled after lunch from 1:00 p.m. to 4:00 p.m., giving her three hours of paid work with a 15-minute break. After her third week on the job, her supervisor, Ms. Ryan, informed her that the hours would change and her shift would start at 1:30 and end at 4:30, with a 15-minute break. Angelica had a meltdown at home that night, telling her mom that she wanted to quit her job. When her mom asked why, Angelica told her about the change in her work time, and said that she wanted to quit because it would be too hard for her to work at the new time.

Figure 6.1. PLAN strategy.

After an hour of talking about the change, Angelica was finally able to say that she did not know what she would do from 1:00-1:30 if the bus dropped her off at work at 1:00 and she didn't start work until 1:30.

She also was worried because she usually did her yoga exercise tape at 4:30 after she got home from work, so she could be finished before dinner at 5:30. Her mom told her they would be happy to change dinner to 6:00 p.m. and then reminded her to use the strategy she learned in middle school called, "What's My Plan" (see Figure 6.1). Her mom helped her use the strategy to figure out how to solve the time problem before she went to work.

Using the PLAN Strategy to Build Flexibility

Young adults with flexibility have the ability to understand and accept the need to change their perceptions, feelings, thoughts, and actions based on the current situation (McCloskey & Perkins, 2013). However, many students with autism who are transitioning from high school to adult life are faced with problems that seem insurmountable, and they often feel "stuck" with no solution or next steps to move on from the problem. This lack of flexibility prevents them from moving forward when faced with obstacles, mistakes, or new information. The *PLAN Strategy* is a step-by-step process for solving both small and large problems.

 Why Is This Important?

PLAN provides a visual support to guide students through a problem-solving structure that increases flexibility by identifying whether there is a problem, finding possible solutions to the problem, choosing the best solution, and ultimately building independence in future problem solving (Sam et al., 2015). PLAN also supports *Predictors of Successful Secondary Transition* outcomes related to self-determination/self-advocacy (NTACT, 2015).

Teacher Directions: When and How to Use PLAN

Stage 1 Learners

For Stage One learners, introduce the PLAN process by defining and giving examples for each of the four steps (see Figure 6.2). Go over the sample *What's My PLAN* chart (see Figure 6.3). Guide a discussion about the steps and solutions (replace with an age-appropriate example for younger students). Lead group practice by presenting familiar problems, guiding students to voice solutions, and model by filling out a poster-size *What's My PLAN* chart (see Figure 6.3, Appendix E). Encourage and reinforce participation, while sharing and building on student ideas.

Stage 2 Learners

For Stage Two learners, introduce the *PLAN Strategy* by reviewing each PLAN step (see Figure 6.2). Model filling out the *What's My PLAN* chart (see Figure 6.3) using the sample situation. Talk about one or two additional real or hypothetical situations and use a poster size PLAN chart, having students take turns writing the information on the chart to build flexible thinking skills. Have students work in groups of two to practice filling out their own *What's My PLAN* chart (see Figure 6.3), using real or suggested problems.

Stage 3 Learners

For Stage Three Learners, guide regular practice using the *What's My PLAN* chart (see Figure 6.3) at least once a week to support students as they practice and become independent at using flexible thinking with PLAN to solve their problems. Have the *PLAN Steps* on display as a poster and refer to the steps as real problems arise during the school week, involving individual or groups of students in the problem-solving process. (See *Directions for Students* below.)

PLAN Steps

Step 1: P = Is there a Problem?
- Is this situation causing stress and anxiety and/or keeping you from moving forward? If "yes," this **is** a problem for you.

Step 2: L = Is it a Little Problem or a Big Problem?
- Ask yourself, is there a simple solution to solve this problem that involves no more than one or two steps and does not involve more than one other person? If "yes," this is most likely a **little problem**.
- If the solution is more than two steps, involves two or more people, and takes time and/or resources to solve, it is probably a **big problem**.
- Note: If you or someone else is in a situation that is hurtful, dangerous, or causing damage, it is a **BIG problem** and you should get help right away.

Step 3: A = What is my Plan A & Plan B?
- Plan A may be the first thing you do when faced with a problem. It is important to think of at least one more possible solution that you could do if Plan A does not work.

Step 4: N = What is my Next step?
- Once you have figured out a Plan A and Plan B, decide which will work best and implement the plan.

Figure 6.2. PLAN Steps for problem solving.

What's My PLAN?	
PLAN	**Answers and Solutions**
P = Is there a Problem?	Yes, work shift time changed – not sure what to do when arriving 30 minutes early
L = Is it Little or Big?	Little = What do I do from 1:00-1:30?
A = Plan A and Plan B?	Plan A – quit my job, lose school credit and money Plan B – work at the new time, arrive early, and find a quiet place to do homework or listen to music until my shift starts
N = Next step?	Angelica chose Plan B and was happy she had time to get most of her homework done before work started.

Figure 6.3. What's My PLAN chart for problem solving–example.

Directions for Students

When and How to Use PLAN

Solving big and little problems is important at home, at school, and on the job. First, you need to know when you actually have a problem. Sometimes it's hard to know, so you need to pay attention to a few things like the examples below:

- Your teacher or boss tells you to do something differently and they might seem mad.
- People at school or work are acting different or weird with you.
- Something you are trying to do seems really confusing.

Once you know you have a problem, use the four *PLAN Steps* to solve your problem (Figure 6.2):

1. P= Is there a problem? If there is a problem, go on to the next step.
2. L= Is it a little or a big problem? Decide if this is a really big problem or something pretty small. If it's not something you can ignore, go on to the next step.
3. A= Come up with two options to solve the problem- Plan A or Plan B. If you are having a hard time coming up with at least two solutions, it's a good idea to ask your parent, teacher, or a friend for some ideas.
4. N=What is your next step? Once you have two or more solutions, choose one and see if it works. If it doesn't work, go through the *PLAN Steps* again.

Remember, by knowing when you have a problem, and then solving the problem, you are advocating for yourself.

Data Collection

Use the *PLAN Data Collection* sheet (see Figure 6.4, Appendix E) to record how the student uses the *PLAN Strategy*. Document the type of problem encountered, whether or not the student used the PLAN steps/skills, and if the student initiated the strategy or needed direct or indirect prompts. The example below shows how Angelica used the *PLAN Strategy* successfully to solve two of the three problems documented on the data tool (see Figure 6.4).

PLAN Data Collection				
Student: *Angelica*				
Directions: For each problem listed, describe whether the student used the PLAN Steps and, if so, whether the problem was solved.				
Date:	**Describe the Problem**		**Used PLAN Steps: Y/N**	**Problem Solved: Y/N**
11/5	Work shift changed		☑ yes ☐ no	☑ yes ☐ no
11/10	New job tasks assigned on new shift		☐ yes ☑ no	☐ yes ☑ no
11/14	New job tasks are too hard (I want to quit)		☑ yes ☐ no	☑ yes ☐ no
			☐ yes ☐ no	☐ yes ☐ no
			☐ yes ☐ no	☐ yes ☐ no

Figure 6.4. PLAN strategy data collection tool–example.

Leveled Emotions: *Visual Scale Strategy*

Many students with ASD have concrete thought processes and interpret information literally, which can cause confusion when communicating with others, especially in new situations. A young adult transitioning from the supportive high school environment to postsecondary education or employment may need support to understand and cope with new social situations.

A *Visual Scale* can be helpful in understanding and controlling anxiety by allowing the individual to identify how he is feeling and then use a calming strategy to self-regulate. *Visual Scales* have been used effectively with all age groups as illustrations of social behaviors, abstract ideas, and emotions (Coffin & Smith, 2009). This visual support allows the young adult to build independence by monitoring his/her own behavior (Sam et al., 2015) and acts as an antecedent-based intervention by providing a visual prompt that prevents negative behavior from occurring (Sam et al., 2016a).

In an educational or work situation, a *Visual Scale* can be used to identify anxiety and dysregulation and allow the young adult to gain control and self-regulate. The *Visual Scale* will demonstrate how abstract concepts can be broken into concrete parts (Buron & Curtis, 2012). For example, the levels of anxiety or dysregulation the person is feeling are not "off" or "on," but fall on a scale that moves gradually in steps from low to high. A typical *Visual Scale* is one that is created with the numbers from 1 to 5, with 1 representing low anxiety and 5 representing high anxiety (see Figure 6.5).

5-Point Scale		
	How I am feeling:	**What I need to do:**
5	I am totally anxious and stressed; my heart is racing; I am breathing very fast; I can't sit still.	**Take a break and ask for help.**
4	I am feeling really anxious and stressed; my heartbeat and breathing are getting fast.	**Take a short walk.**
3	I am starting to feel anxious and stressed; my heartbeat is a little fast.	**Use deep breathing app.**
2	I'm a little anxious but my body is calm.	**Take action and I'll be OK.**
1	I am feeling calm.	**Keep doing what I'm doing.**

Figure 6.5. 5-point scale for self-regulation.

Why Is This Important?

The function of a *Visual Scale* is to help the young adult be aware of and identify his emotional and physical state. *Visual Scales* can be developed to meet the specific needs of the student and to address specific skills, such as their work schedule. Checking the scale on a regular basis throughout the day will allow the person to better predict when circumstances and events have had an impact and may affect self-regulation.

Teacher Directions: When and How to Use the *Visual Scale*

A *Visual Scale*, as shown in Figure 6.5, may be personalized for each student to fit specific situations, then photocopied on card stock and laminated. *Visual Scales* can also be stored on a phone or tablet as a photo that can be easily found and used as a quick reference for the young adult.

Stage 1 Learners   For Stage One Learners, introduce the *Visual Scale* process by describing a difficult situation at school that may cause anxiety or dysregulation, such as:

- Not understanding the assignment after the teacher explained and said to figure it out.
- Being teased and shoved during break/recess.
- An unexpected change in the schedule that caused you to miss your break.

Next, model how a student might feel or react to the sample situation and then go over the scale to describe the five levels in the scale and how each would be used by a student (see Figure 6.5). Give each student a personalized *Visual Scale* to keep in their desk, binder, or device. Teach the levels by guiding and prompting students to recognize when to use the scale, and then reinforcing their use of the scale.

Stage 2 Learners   For Stage Two learners, introduce the *Visual Scale* as described above and then talk about one or two additional real or hypothetical situations using the *Visual Scale* to increase practice and build self-regulation skills. Have students design their own *Visual Scale*, using information from the *5-Point Scale* (see Figure 6.5) and personalizing the columns, "how I am feeling," and "what I need to do." Students then role play, using their personalized scale.

Stage 3 Learners   For Stage Three Learners, students practice using their personalized *Visual Scale* (see activity to personalize the *5-Point Scale in Directions for Students* below). Hold discussions with individuals or small groups of students to talk about real and simulated situations and how to use their *Visual Scale*. Check-in with students on a weekly basis to go over situations in which they used or should have use their *Visual Scale* and offer suggestions for future use. Be sure to reinforce students for use of the *Visual Scale* in real time.

Directions for Students

When and How to Use Your *Visual Scale*

We can all feel anxious, scared, or dysregulated when we go into new or unexpected situations. When this happens, you can get back in control by using the *Visual Scale* strategy.

The *5-Point Scale* is a great strategy that you can personalize just for you! You can talk to your teacher to be sure you know what each of the five levels mean. You can identify your level of regulation in different situations and then apply it to the scale. You will use the five levels of the *Visual Scale* throughout the day – your teacher may remind you to use the scale or may support you by asking, "What's your level?"

It's also a good idea to debrief with your teacher so you can identify the levels, from when you are regulated to when you are not regulated, and the best strategies to use with each level. Remember, by using the *Visual Scale*, you can be in control of your emotions and stay self-regulated.

Data Collection

After teaching, modeling, and having students practice using the *Visual Scale*, guide students to monitor their own use of the *Visual Scale* by keeping data on the *Visual Scale Data Collection* sheet (see Figure 6.6, Appendix E). In the example below, Angelica was able to reduce her anxiety at work over the five days (see Figure 6.6).

Visual Scale Data Collection					
Level of Emotion: *(See the 5-Point Scale)*	**5 Extremely Anxious** Take break and ask for help	**4 Really Anxious** Take short walk	**3 Anxious** Use deep breathing app	**2 Calm to Anxious** Take action and I'll be OK	**1 Calm & OK** Keep doing what I'm doing

Name: Angelica		**Place:**	❑ **Home**	❑ **School**	☑ **Work**

Directions: Pick one place (home, school, work) and keep track of your emotions for five days by using your *Visual Scale*.

Date: 11/10	My level of emotion was: 5	I used the Visual Scale: ☑ yes ❑ no	I reduced my anxiety: ❑ yes ☑ no	If no, what will I do next time: *Only took break- will also ask for help*
Date: 11/11	My level of emotion was: 5	I used the Visual Scale: ☑ yes ❑ no	I reduced my anxiety: ❑ yes ☑ no	If no, what will I do next time: *Need to ask for help sooner*
Date: 11/12	My level of emotion was: 5	I used the Visual Scale: ☑ yes ❑ no	I reduced my anxiety: ☑ yes ❑ no	If no, what will I do next time: *Need to take a walk sooner*
Date: 11/13	My level of emotion was: 3	I used the Visual Scale: ☑ yes ❑ no	I reduced my anxiety: ☑ yes ❑ no	If no, what will I do next time: *Need to use deep breathing app*
Date: 11/14	My level of emotion was: 2	I used the Visual Scale: ☑ yes ❑ no	I reduced my anxiety: ☑ yes ❑ no	If no, what will I do next time:

Figure 6.6. Visual scale data collection–example.

Impulse Control: *Job Interview Reminder Card Strategy*

Interviewing for a job is usually stressful for anyone. It can be especially challenging for students who struggle with impulse control and have a tendency to interrupt others or answer questions without thinking about their response.

A job interview reminder card is a visual cue, individualized for this specific situation, created and placed on a piece of paper, an index card, business card, or other media (e.g., smartphone) that is easily accessible. It can be an effective tool in giving reminders on what behavior is expected during a job interview and in helping to control impulses.

Why Is This Important?

The function of the *Tips for Job Interviews Card* is to give the young adult a reminder of the behavior that is expected during a job interview.

> **Tips for Job Interviews**
>
> 1. **Greet your interviewer**
>   - Make eye contact.
>   - Say hello.
>   - Shake hands.
> 2. **Listen attentively** to questions and ask for clarification if you don't understand something.
> 3. **Answer** each question to the best of your ability.
> 4. **Be aware** of any nervous habits you have and:
>   - Monitor nervous habits.
>   - Relax and be calm.
>   - Be yourself.
> 5. **Say "Thank you"** at the end of the interview.

Figure 6.7. Job interview reminder card.

The reminder card also serves to help the young adult prepare for the interview and then use the five tips to monitor and control her impulses during the interview.

Teacher Directions: When and How to Use the *Tips for Job Interviews Card*

Stage 1 Learners

For Stage One learners, use a poster size visual of the *Tips for Job Interviews Card,* along with small copies for each student. Go over each of the five tips (Figure 6.7), modeling and demonstrating each behavior. Also show what it looks like when you are not using those behaviors to give students both good examples and bad or non-examples, (e.g., looking at the floor, laughing, mumbling, flapping). Have students practice in pairs and critique each other. For example, for Tip #2, use simple questions such as:

1. What is your favorite subject in school? Why?
2. What type of activity (or job) do you like best? Why?
3. What skill would you like to learn or improve? Why?

Stage 2 Learners

For Stage Two learners, after teaching the skill (see Stage One Learner examples), create simulated situations for students to practice. It is effective to have other staff assist by taking the role of interviewer during practice sessions to ensure students are learning and practicing the five tips for job interviews (see Figure 6.7).

Stage 3 Learners

For Stage Three learners, guide students to make their own portable *Tips for Job Interviews Card* as a business-size card or 3 x 5 index card to practice and role-play with partners. Students can also make the *Reminder Card* in a digital format for use on a tablet, smartphone or other device. Once students have practiced using the five tips, arrange to videotape interview sessions and then sit with the student to view and critique the session. (See *Directions for Students* below.)

Directions for Students

When and How to Use the *Job Interview Card*

Going to a job interview can cause most of us to feel anxious, nervous, and scared. One way to reduce these feelings is to prepare. The *Job Interview Card* is a strategy to guide the preparation process.

Use the *Job Interview Card* to prepare for the interview by practicing with friends and family. Prior to a job interview, review the information on the card. You can do this at home for several days prior to the job interview, before you leave on the day of the interview, and immediately prior to the interview. The job reminder card can be placed in your wallet for quick reference or created on a mobile device. After each interview (practice or real) take data to determine areas in which you did well and areas where you need to improve.

Remember, by using the *Job Interview Card*, you can be in control of your emotions and stay self-regulated!

Data Collection

Assist the student to set up interviews for both practice and real situations, if possible. Review and model using the *Interview Data Collection Worksheet* (Figure 6.8, Appendix E) with the student, individually or in a small group. This example shows how Angelica improved her interviewing skills with different interviewers over four weeks (see Figure 6.8).

Interview Data Collection Worksheet					
Student: Angelica					
Directions: • Write the name of the interviewer. • Write the date of the interview. • Score yourself on each of the six behaviors. • Add up your scores. • Continue to practice skills with scores of 1 and 0 points.		**Scoring Key:** Yes-Did it well = 2 OK-Sometimes = 1 No-Not at all = 0			
Interviewer(s): Ms. Taylor, Career Center Mr. Stein, Math Teacher, Ms. Allen, Office Mrs. Vasquez, Cafeteria Supervisor	**Date:** 11/5	**Date:** 11/12	**Date:** 11/19	**Date:** 12/5	**Date:**
1. Greeted the Interviewer: made eye contact, shook hands, said hello.	1	2	2	2	
2. Looked at and listened to the interviewer.	1	1	2	2	
3. Asked questions when I didn't understand something.	0	1	1	1	
4. Answered each question to the best of my ability.	1	1	1	2	
5. Looked at the interviewer and gave eye contact a few times during my answers.	2	2	2	2	
6. Said "thank you" at the end of the interview.	2	1	2	2	
Mastery = 10 -12 points. **Total:**	7	8	10	11	
Comments: Working on eye contact and knowing my answers.					

Figure 6.8. Interview data collection tool for students–example.

Planning and Organizing: *Career Search Portfolio Strategy*

When looking for employment, the executive function skill of planning and organizing is a key component for a successful outcome. Planning and organizing a job search includes preparing information about the young adult student, as well as information about potential jobs. The *Career Search Portfolio* is a strategy that will assist the young adult student through this process. The first step is to organize a visual representation of the student's qualifications, skills, and experiences, including important information and documents. The next step is to develop a network of people who can provide information and job leads to support a job search. Fulton and Silva (2018) developed a set of "New Modern Methods" for job searches that focus on "networking," rather than the traditional "help wanted" advertisements. Using this method, students develop a list of networking contacts who can provide information about possible job leads, or help the student "get their foot in the door," by assisting with setting up things such as job shadowing, volunteering, and other activities that might turn into future jobs.

To complete the first step in the process, the young adult student will create a *Career Search Portfolio* to organize their information in a binder or folder, using tabs and page protectors. This information can also be scanned and managed as an electronic version to be used in an online employment process. When compiled and presented in a clear and concise manner, the *Career Search Portfolio* can show a potential employer the student's organizational skills and attention to detail. The portfolio can also be used in the preparation process for a job interview, as the student can review the information, giving her confidence to answer interview questions about her skills, strengths, education, and experience.

 Why Is This Important?

A *Career Search Portfolio* can assist students in planning and organizing information needed to do a job search. The *Career Search Portfolio* will help organize and keep track of documents that are relevant to a job search. It will also organize and guide the job search process through the networking steps.

Teacher Directions: When and How to Use the *Career Search Portfolio*

All Learners
For all learners, prepare a sample Career Search Portfolio binder organized with sample documents listed in the *Career Search Portfolio Guide* (Figure 6.9). Review the purpose of the binder and explain each of the documents and how they would be used for a job search, when completing a job application process. Guide students to make their own *Career Search Portfolio*. The portfolio will provide easy access to the documents the student will need for job applications and interviews, such as a resumé and letters of recommendation. Guide the student to put together the portfolio, as described in the section *Career Search Portfolio Guide* (Figure 6.9). The last document in the portfolio is the *Networking Worksheet* (see Figure 6.11, Appendix E). Once the other components are ready, review the *Steps for Networking* (see Figure 6.10) and the *Networking Worksheet – Example* (see Figure 6.11) and have students fill out the form as part of their career search (see *Directions for Students* below).

Career Search Portfolio Guide
Student Directions: Separate each section using labeled divider tabs. Use plastic sheet protectors to store documents, adding multiple copies of documents such as resumé, letters of recommendation, transcripts, and certificates.
❏ **Personal Information**—Add a sheet with your name, address, phone, email, and emergency contacts.
❏ **Resumé**—Place several copies of your updated resumé in this section.
❏ **Letters of Recommendation**—Add several copies of each letter. These can be from former employers, teachers, or supervisors of volunteer activities, who will write a letter to draw attention to skills you have that would make you a good employee.
❏ **References**—Add a reference list of three to five people who would be willing to talk about your abilities and expertise. Include their name, title, address, and email/phone number. Be sure to ask the people on your list ahead of time if it is okay to use their name as a reference.
❏ **Education and Training**—Add several copies of high school transcripts, degrees, relevant coursework, and certifications of technical training or other training you may have completed.
❏ **Cover Page**—Create a cover page and place inside the plastic see-through cover on the binder.
❏ **Networking Worksheet**—Place a copy of completed *Networking Worksheet(s)* (Figure 6.10) in this section. Use this to keep track of information related to the jobs you are interested in, as well as your job application submissions, interview details including names of personnel you met during interviews, and the date you followed up with the company.

Figure 6.9. Career search portfolio guide for students.

Steps for Networking	
Make a Network List	<u>Make a Network List</u> of friends and family and everyone else you know who might have connections that will help in your job search. Ask for help to make your list from your parents and teachers.
Ask for Job Leads and Contacts	Call the people on your Network List and ask for job leads. <u>Get a contact name </u>and phone number for each job lead and write this on your Career Search Portfolio.
Research All Job Leads	Use the internet and the people from your network list to <u>research each of your job leads</u>. Get information about the company and write this information on your *Career Search Portfolio.*
List Questions to Ask Job Leads	Think about the information you have about the job lead. <u>Make a set of four to five questions</u> you can ask when you call the job lead contact.
Call the Job Lead Contact	Call each job lead contact to ask questions. <u>Keep notes from the call</u> in the *Career Search Portfolio.*
Prepare to Answer Questions about YOU	Before each call, <u>prepare for an informal interview</u>. The job lead contact may be interested in you and will ask questions to see if you would be a good employee for their company.
Follow-up With a Thank You Note	Be sure you have the address for your job lead contact and <u>follow up with a short thank you note</u>.

Figure 6.10. Steps for networking–student directions (adapted from Fulton & Silva, 2018).

Networking Worksheet			
Name: Angelica		**Date:**	

	Name		**Phone Number**
Make a Network List • Names of Family & Friends • Phone Numbers • Ask for job contacts	Dad–John Vasquez		(000) 222-2222
	Aunt– Leslie Smith		(000) 221-2221
	Friend– Tim Jones		(000) 223-2223
	Neighbor– Amber Green		(000) 224-2224
	Teacher– Sue Craft		(000) 225-2225

	Contact Name & Company		**Phone Number**
List Job Lead Contacts • Names of Contact & Company • Phone Numbers	Jim Smith, ABC School District		(000) 333-3333
	Jane Lance, One Bank		(000) 332-3332
	Alex Sanders, Ace Insurance		(000) 334-3334
	Victor Stein, Jumper USA		(000) 335-3335
	Jones, Best Craft		(000) 336-3336

	Company A	**Company B**	**Company C**
Select 3 Companies & Jobs to Research • Company facts • What they do • Jobs you would like	One Bank Main 444 Ball Street Banking savings, loans, filing, typing Teller, Clerk	Ace Insurance 333 First Street, Insurance policies, filing typing Office Clerk	Fitness USA Center 444 8th & 1212 Bailey Gym memberships & floor workouts Front Desk clerk
List Questions to Ask about– • Job openings • Requirements for jobs–education & experience • Advice for a potential job candidate	Are there openings for tellers or clerks? What are the requirements for tellers and clerks? What should I do to get a job here?	Are there openings for office clerks? What are the requirements? What training or experience is needed?	Are there openings for front desk clerks? What are the requirements for front desk clerks? What should I have to work here?
Call the Contact • Write date of call	October 20	October 30	November 1
Send Thank You • Write date sent	October 22	October 31	November 2
Prepare to Answer Questions	Review your *Career Search Portfolio* and have it in front of you when you make the call. When you are asked questions, you can refer to information in the portfolio.		

Figure 6.11. Networking worksheet–example.

Directions for Students

How to Use Your *Career Search Portfolio*

Follow directions in the section *Career Search Portfolio Guide* (see Figure 6.8). Have someone look over your portfolio to make sure it is error-free. If you have a computer, you can create a folder and keep scanned copies of the documents that are in your portfolio.

- Practice presenting the information from your portfolio to family or friends. This is good preparation for a job interview, as some questions will be related to what is in your portfolio.
- Remember to take your portfolio to your job interviews. Set it down next to you when you are seated after greeting the interviewer. Make extra copies and be ready to give copies of documents to the interviewer if they ask, such as your resume' and letters of recommendation. Do not force the portfolio on the interviewer.
- Remember to update your portfolio when information changes, including new skills, training, experience, and other accomplishments.
- It's a good idea to take your portfolio to your first day of work, as you may need to verify or provide personal information you have listed in your portfolio.

Remember to complete the *Networking Worksheet* (Figure 6.10, see Appendix E) using the *Steps for Networking* (see Figure 6.9) for more information. This is an important tool that will guide your career search.

 Data Collection

The completed *Career Search Portfolio* and *Networking Worksheet* (see Figure 6.11, Appendix E) serve as data for this strategy. In the previous example (see Figure 6.11), Angelica makes lists of people for networking and for job leads. She also selects three potential employers to research. The *Networking Worksheet* provides a structure for Angelica to begin her career search.

Problem Solving: *SOARR Strategy*

Angelica was feeling anxious at work every time she had to work in the office to check the inventory lists of items she stocked that day. The office had ten desks and computers, and employees could use any computer, once they logged in to their account. There were at least ten people in a shift, and there were always coworkers at three or four computers. Angelica liked to use the computer in the corner farthest from the window because there was less noise and glare. But sometimes that computer was taken, making her feel anxious and unsure of what to do. The last time this happened she went back to the sales floor and then had to stay after work for 30 minutes to do her inventory documentation. Ms. Brock, her job coach, helped her analyze the problem using SOARR (see Figure 6.12).

SOARR Chart				
Specify	**Observe**	**Analyze**	**Respond**	**Reflect**
What is the context or specific situation?	What do I see in this situation? How are other people behaving?	What do I need to do to fit in to this situation? What questions do I need to ask and answer in my head?	Based on my analysis of the situation, what did I do?	What happened? What did I learn? What will I do differently next time?
My usual computer is not open for me to use. I need to find an open computer in the office to complete my work.	Co-workers are sitting at 5 of the 10 computers. They are working and making comments to each other.	I need to get my work done. Where is the best place for me to work? Is there an open computer is in a quiet place with no glare from the window? Is it OK to talk quietly to my co-workers while I'm working if I have a question or they ask me a question?	First, I took 3 deep breaths and then looked for an open computer in a quiet area. My co-workers didn't pay attention to me, so I felt OK walking around the room. I found a computer in the corner with no glare and I was able to get my work done.	Even though I felt anxious and self-conscious walking around the office, no one paid attention to me and I was able to relax and find a good spot. The next time this happens, I'll take deep breaths and find another open computer.

Figure 6.12. SOARR chart–example.

SOARR: Specify, Observe, Analyze, Respond and Reflect

The *SOARR Strategy* guides students through a problem-solving process that helps the student identify, respond, and reflect on problems. SOARR is especially effective when used before an expected event or problem situation occurs, thereby increasing opportunities to build flexible thinking and problem-solving skills. SOARR also allows the young adult to reflect on the situation after it has happened.

SOARR can be used in a variety of situations to build problem-solving skills and increase flexibility for young adults transitioning from school to adult life. These skills lead to increased self-determination/self-advocacy, an outcome for successful transition from school to adult life (NTACT, 2015). Examples include:

- Actively participating in the IEP
- Participating in a group discussion in a general education class
- Buying lunch and eating with peers on campus
- Attending an after-school game or sports activity
- Attending a club or school activity meeting
- Completing a job-shadow experience
- Riding the bus or other public transportation
- Purchasing food or other items at a store

 Why Is This Important?

The *SOARR Strategy* supports students through a problem-solving structure that increases flexibility and self-management by identifying the problem, analyzing the situation, making a response choice, and assessing their response to the situation (Sam et al., 2016b). As such, the process allows the student to build contextual awareness and develop metacognitive skills that will generalize to other situations (Wilkins & Burmeister, 2015).

Teacher Directions: When and How to Use the SOARR Strategy

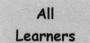

All Learners

Introduce the SOARR process to a small group of young adults by going over each of the prompts on a poster sized *SOARR Chart* (see Figure 6.12, Appendix E). Next, use a relevant sample situation to illustrate each step, charting responses on each section on the SOARR template. Have students take turns presenting a situation and then ask the group to volunteer responses. Remind students to use SOARR when situations arise at school. Debrief with the group at least once per week to review situations in which students did or could have used SOARR. Reinforce all attempts at using the SOARR process (see *Directions for Students* below).

Directions for Students

How to Use the SOARR Strategy

Problems can be overwhelming, especially when they are unexpected. It's a good idea to stay calm by having a quick way to come up with solutions for your problem.

SOARR is a strategy you can use when you have a problem on the job, at home, or in the community. SOARR is a way to figure out the exact problem, and then find and use the best solution. Use the steps from the SOARR chart to:

- Figure out the REAL problem you need to solve by staying calm and looking at the situation.
- Ask yourself questions about the situation to analyze it or figure out what to do.
- Once you figure out what to do, take action or respond to the situation.
- Think about what happened and decide if you had a good response.

SOARR gives you a strategy to stay calm, figure out what's wrong and what do about it. Then you can decide what you have learned from the situation.

Data Collection

Collect class data on how students use the SOARR process, using the *SOARR Data Collection* sheet (see Figure 6.13, Appendix E). In the example below, four students used the *SOARR Strategy* for various problems. The data indicates Angelica, RJ, and Jack have successfully solved their problems (see Figure 6.13).

SOARR Data Collection				
Date	Student Name	Describe the Problem	Used SOARR Strategy? Y/N	Solved Problem? Y/N
11/2	Angelica	Finding a computer in the office to do my work	☑ yes ☐ no	☑ yes ☐ no
11/5	RJ	Noisy areas during passing periods	☑ yes ☐ no	☑ yes ☐ no
11/5	Amiko	Working in a group to do the semester science project	☑ yes ☐ no	☐ yes ☑ no
11/10	Jack	Getting homework done and turned in on time	☑ yes ☐ no	☑ yes ☐ no
			☐ yes ☐ no	☐ yes ☐ no

Figure 6.13. SOARR class data collection sheet–example.

FLIPP 2.0: Making a Difference for Today and Tomorrow

This book has presented a great deal of information regarding evidence-based practices and executive function skills and has introduced numerous strategies that can be used by educators to support the development of EF skills in students with autism. These strategies are developed to support students in building stronger EF skills that are needed throughout the life span.

Too often students with autism leave the educational environment lacking the skills needed to succeed in adult life. Having become dependent on the intervention and support of caring educators, they struggle to succeed when those supports are no longer available to them. Unfortunately, although these young people want to do well at work, in the community, and in social situations, they may have insufficient EF skills to accomplish their goals.

It is not enough to use evidence-based practices with students with autism, hoping that they will somehow realize that they need to implement these practices themselves. We have a responsibility to model the use of these powerful educational strategies, give students plenty of opportunities to practice using them in controlled environments, and provide coaching and continued support as they use the practices in new and unique circumstances. In doing so, we are giving our students an incredible gift that can follow them throughout their lives.

It is our sincere hope that you will find the strategies outlined in this book helpful as you seek to provide your students with autism with the tools they need to succeed once they leave school. We wish you and your students all the very best in the future.

REFERENCES

Alber, S. R., Heward, W. L., & Hippler, B. J. (1999). Teaching middle school students with learning disabilities to recruit positive teacher attention. *Exceptional Children, 64,* 253-270.

Alexander, J. L., Ayres, K. M., & Smith, K. A. (2015). Training teachers in evidence-based practice for individuals with autism spectrum disorder: A review of the literature. *Teacher Education and Special Education, 38*(1), 13-27.

Archer, A.A., & Hughes, C.A. (2011). *Explicit Instruction: Effective and Efficient Teaching.* New York, NY: Guilford Press.

Aspy, R., & Grossman, B.G. (2007). *The Ziggurat Model: A framework for designing comprehensive interventions for individuals with high-functioning autism and Asperger syndrome.* Shawnee Missions, KS: Autism Asperger Publishing Company.

Aspy, R. & Grossman, B.G. (2012). *The Ziggurat Model (2nd ed.).* Shawnee Mission, KS: Autism Asperger Publishing Company.

Barrett, P., Zhang, Y., Davies, F., & Barrett, L. (2015). *Clever classrooms: Summary findings of the HEAD Project (Holistic Evidence and Design).* Salford, UK: University of Salford, Manchester.

Barshay, J. (2018). Does a lack of executive function explain why some kids fall way behind in school? *The Hechinger Report.* Retrieved from http://hechingerreport.org/does-a-lack-of-executive-function-explain-why-some-kids-fall-way-behind-in-school/

Broden, M., Bruce, C., Mitchell, M.A., Carter, V., & Hall, R.V. (1970). Effects of teacher attention on attending behavior of two boys at adjacent desks. *Journal of Applied Behavior Analysis, 3,* 205-211.

Browning Wright, D. (2011, May). *Pacing, structuring, and transitioning for students with autism and behavior problems.* Presentation at the 32nd Annual National Institute on Legal Issues of Educating Individuals with Disabilities, Phoenix, AZ.

Bucholz, J. L., & Sheffler, J. L. (2009). Creating a warm and inclusive classroom environment: Planning for all children to feel welcome. *Electronic Journal for Inclusive Education, 2*(4).

Burkhartsmeyer, J. (2007, May). *Cognitive Characteristics of Children with Autism: Implications for Assessment and Programming.* Presentation for the Region 10 Coordinating Council, Apple Valley, CA.

Buron, K. D., & Curtis, M. (2012). *The incredible 5-point scale: Assisting students with autism spectrum disorders in understanding social interactions and controlling their emotional responses* (2nd ed.). Shawnee Mission, KS: AAPC Publishing.

Buron, K.D., & Myles, B.S. (2014). Emotional Regulation. In K. D. Buron and P. Wolfberg (Eds.) *Learners on the Autism Spectrum: Preparing Highly Qualified Educators and Related Practitioners,* Second Edition (pp. 239-263). Shawnee Mission, KS: AAPC Publishing.

Camacho, R., Anderson, A., Moore, D.W., & Furlonger (2014). Conducting a function-based intervention in a school setting to reduce inappropriate behaviour of a child with autism. *Behaviour Change, 31*(1), 65-77.

Carnahan, C., Hume, K., Clarke, L., & Borders, C. (2009). Using structured work systems to promote independence and engagement for students with autism spectrum disorders. *Teaching Exceptional Children, 41*(4), 6-14.

Carnahan, C., Harte, H., Dyke, K. S., Hume, K., & Borders, C. (2011). Structured work systems: Supporting meaningful engagement in preschool settings for children with autism spectrum disorders. *Young Exceptional Children, 14*(4), 2-16.

Carr, E.G., Dunlap, G., Horner, R.H., Koegel, R.L., Turnbull, A.P., Sailor, W., Anderson, J., Albin, R.W., Koegel, L.K., Fox, L. (2002). Positive behavior support: Evolution of an applied science. *Journal of Positive Behavior Interventions, 4*, 4-16.

Center on the Developing Child at Harvard University. (2014). *Enhancing and practicing executive function skills with children from infancy to adolescence.* Retrieved from www.developingchild.harvard.edu/

Centers for Medicare and Medicaid Services. (2010). Autism spectrum disorders: Final report on environmental scan. Washington, DC: Author.

Chasnoff, I.J. (2010). *The mystery of risk: Drugs, alcohol, pregnancy, and the vulnerable child.* Chicago, IL: NTI Upstream.

Coffin, A. B., & Smith, S. M. (2009). The Incredible 5-point scale: Online training module (Cincinnati, OH: University of Cincinnati, College of Education, Criminal Justice, and Human Services. In Ohio Center for Autism and Low Incidence (OCALI), *Autism Internet Modules*, www.autisminternetmodules.org/

Common Core State Standards Initiative. (2018). English language arts standards. Retrieved from http://www.corestandards.org/wp-content/uploads/ELA_Standards1.pdf

Constable, S., Grosse, B., Moniz, A., and Ryan, L. (2013). Meeting the common core standards for students with autism: The challenge for educators. *Teaching Exceptional Children, 45*(3), 6-13.

Cooper-Kahn, J. & Dietzel, J. (2008). What is executive functioning? Reprint (2017) at www.ldonline.org from Cooper-Kahn, J. & Dietzel, J. (2008). *Late, lost, and unprepared* (pp. 9-14). Bethesda, MD: Woodbine House.

Coyne, P., & Rood, K. (2011). Unit 3.3: Executive function and organization for youth with autism spectrum disorder. In *Preparing youth with autism spectrum disorder for adulthood*. Columbia, OR: Columbia Regional Program. Retrieved from http://impactofspecialneeds.weebly.com/uploads/3/4/1/9/3419723/aut_unit3.3_organization.pdf

Craft, M. A., Alber, S. R., & Heward, W. L. (1998). Teaching elementary students with developmental disabilities to recruit teacher attention in a general education classroom: Effects of teacher praise and academic productivity. *Journal of Applied Behavior Analysis, 31*(3), 399-415.

Dipedeo, A. O., Storlie, C., & Johnson, C. (2015). College students with high-functioning autism spectrum disorder: Best practices for successful transition to the world of work. *Journal of College Counseling, 18*, 175-190.

DiPipi-Hoy, C., & Steere, D. (2016). *Teaching time management to learners with autism spectrum disorder*. Shawnee Mission, KS: AAPC Publishing.

Dunlap, G., Carr, E.G, Horner, R.H., Zarcone, J.R., & Schwartz, I. (2008). Positive behavior support and applied behavior analysis. *Behavior Modification 32*(5), 682-698.

Ellis. E.S. (1989). A metacognitive intervention for increasing class participation. *Learning Disabilities Focus, 5*(1), 36-46.

Ennis, R.P., Royer, D.J., Lane, K.L., & Griffith, C.E. (2017). A systematic review of precorrection in PK-12 settings. *Education and Treatment of Children 40*(4), 465–496.

Ferguson, E., & Houghton, S. (1992). The effects of contingent teacher praise, as specified by Canter's Assertive Discipline Programme, on children's on-task behaviour. *Educational Studies, 1,* 83-93.

Floress, M.T., Beschta, S.L., Meyer, K.L., & Reinke, W.M. (2017). Praise research trends and future directions: Characteristics and teacher training. *Behavioral Disorders 43*(1), 227-243.

Freedman, S. (2010). *Developing college skills in students with autism and Asperger's Syndrome.* London, UK: Jessica Kingsley Publishers.

Fulton, L. & Silva, R. (2018). *The Transitions Curriculum* (4th ed.). Santa Barbara, CA: James Stanfield Company.

Gagnon, E. (2006, January). *Autism and Asperger Syndrome: Classroom strategies that really make a difference! (Grades K-12).* Presentation at the California Elementary Education Association, Ontario, CA.

Gagnon, E. & Myles, B. S. (2016). *Power Card Strategy 2.0: Using special interests to motivate children and youth with Autism Spectrum Disorder.*

Gallow, D. (2015). *Working effectively with small groups.* UCI Center for Engaged Instruction. Retrieved from http://cei.uci.edu/wp-content/uploads/sites/26/2015/12/Working-Effectively-with-Small-Groups-Jan-2016.pdf/

Gawande, A. (2009). *The Checklist Manifesto.* New York, New York: Picador Publishing.

Gerhardt, P. (2017). *Employment and individuals on the autism spectrum*. Autism Society of America. Retrieved from http://www.autism-society.org/news/ask-expert-employment-individuals-autism-spectrum/

Goetz, E. M., Holmberg, M. C., & LeBlanc, J. M. (1975). Differential reinforcement of other behavior and noncontingent reinforcement as control procedures during the modification of a preschooler's compliance. *Journal of Applied Behavior Analysis, 8*(1), 77-82.

Golden, C. (2012). *The special educator's toolkit: Everything you need to organize, manage, and monitor your classroom.* Baltimore, MD: Paul H. Brookes Publishing Co.

Hall, R. V., Fox, R., Willard, D., Goldsmith, L., Emerson, M., Owen, M., Davis, F., & Porcia, E. (1971). The teacher as observer and experimenter in the modification of disputing and talking-out behaviors. *Journal of Applied Behavior Analysis, 4*(2), 141-149.

Hedley, D., Cai, R., Uljarevic, M., Wilmot, M., Spoor, J. R., Richdale, A., & Dissanayake, C. (2017). Transition to work: Perspectives from the autism spectrum. *Autism 22(5),* 1-14.

Henry, K. A. (2005). *How do I teach this kid?* Arlington, TX: Future Horizons.

Henry, S. A., & Myles, B. S. (2013). *The comprehensive autism planning system (CAPS) for individuals with Asperger Syndrome, autism, and related disabilities: Integrating best practices throughout the student's day* (2nd ed.). Shawnee Mission, KS: AAPC Publishing.

Horner, R.H., & Sugai, G. (2015) School-wide PBIS: An example of applied behavior analysis implemented at a scale of social importance. *Behavior Analysis Practice* (8), 80-85.

REFERENCES

Horner, R. H., Sugai, G., & Anderson, C. M. (2010). Examining the evidence base for school-wide positive behavior support. *Focus on Exceptional Children 42*(8), 1-14.

Hume, K. (2010). Effective instructional strategies for students with autism spectrum disorders: Keys to enhancing literacy instruction. In C. Carnahan & P. Williamson (Eds.), *Quality literacy instruction for students with autism spectrum disorders* (pp. 45-84). Shawnee Mission, KS: AAPC Publishing.

Hume, K. (2013). *Visual supports (VS) fact sheet.* Chapel Hill, NC: The University of North Carolina, Frank Porter Graham Child Development Institute, the National Professional Development Center on Autism Spectrum Disorders.

Hume, K., & Odom, S. (2007). Effects of an individual work system on the independent functioning of students with autism. *Journal of Autism and Developmental Disorders 37*(6), 1166-80.

Hume, K., & Reynolds, B. (2010). Implementing work systems across the school day: Increasing engagement in students with ASD. *Preventing School Failure, 54,* 228- 227.

Individuals with Disabilities Education Act, 20 U.S.C § 1400 (2004).

Johnson, C, & Ruiter, G. (2013). (Re)-Envisioning classroom design with light and colour. *Academic Research International, 4* (4), 551-559.

Kennedy, M. J., Peeples, K. N., Romig, J. E., Mathews, H. M., & Rodgers, W. J. (2018). *Welcome to our new series on high-leverage practices for students with disabilities.* https://highleverage-practices.org/701-2-2/.

Kern, L., & Clemens, N. (2007). Antecedent strategies to promote appropriate classroom behavior. *Psychology in Schools, 44*(1), 65-75.

Koyama, T. & Wang, Hui-Ting. (2011). Use of activity schedule to promote independent performance of individuals with autism and other intellectual disabilities: A review. *Research in Developmental Disabilities 32* (6), 2235-2242. Retrieved from http://www.northwestaba.com/uploads/7/5/5/1/7551608/koyama11_a_review_of_activity_schedule.pdf

Lewis, T.J., Hudson, S., Richter, M., & Johnson, N. (2004). Scientifically supported practices in emotional and behavioral disorders: A proposed approach and brief review of current practices. *Behavioral Disorders, 29,* 247-259.

Liaupsin, C. J., & Cooper, J. T. (2017). Function-based intervention plans: What and how to teach. *Beyond Behavior, 26*(3), 135-140.

McClannahan, L., & Krantz, P. (2010). *Activity schedules for children with autism: Teaching independent behavior* (2nd ed.). Bethesda, MD: Woodbine House, Inc.

McCloskey, G., & Perkins, L. A., (2013). *Essentials of executive functions assessment.* Hoboken, NJ: John Wiley & Sons, Inc.

Marchant, M., & Anderson, D. H. (2012). Improving the social and academic outcomes for all learners through the use of teacher praise. *Beyond Behavior, 21*(3), 22-28.

Marder, T., & deBettencourt, L. (2015). Teaching students with ASD using evidence-based practices: Why is training critical now? *Teacher Education and Special Education, 38*(1), 5-12.

Mataya, K., & Owens, P. (2013). *Successful problem solving for high functioning students with autism spectrum disorders.* Shawnee Mission, KS: AAPC Publishing.

Meier. D. (2013, April 11). Explaining KIPP's SLANT (blog post). *Education Week.* Retrieved from http://blogs.edweek.org/edweek/Bridging-Differences/2013/04/slant_and_the_golden_rule. html

Mesibov, G. B., & Shea, V. (2014). Structured teaching and environmental supports. In K. D. Buron & P. Wolfberg (Eds.), *Learners on the autism spectrum: Preparing highly qualified educators and related practitioners* (2nd ed., pp. 264-287). Shawnee Mission, KS: AAPC Publishing.

Mesibov, G., Shea, V., & Schopler, E. (2005). *The TEACCH approach to autism spectrum disorders*. New York, NY: Plenum Press.

Minshew, N.J. & Williams, D.L. (2008). Brain-behavior connections in autism. In K.D. Buron & P. Wolfberg (Eds.), *Learners on the autism spectrum: Preparing highly qualified educators* (pp. 45-65). Shawnee Mission, Kansas: Autism Asperger Publishing Co.

Mussey, J., Dawkins, T., & AFIRM Team. (2017). *Cognitive behavioral intervention*. Chapel Hill, NC: National Professional Development Center on Autism Spectrum Disorder, FPG Child Development Center, University of North Carolina. Retrieved from http://afirm.fpg.unc.edu/cognitive-behavioral-intervention.

Myles, B. S., Aspy, R., Mataya, K., & Shaffer, J. (2018). *Excelling with autism: Obtaining critical mass using deliberate practice*. Shawnee Mission, KS: AAPC Publishing.

National Autism Center. (2015). *Findings and conclusions: National Standards Project, phase 2*. Randolph, MA: Author.

National Technical Assistance Center on Transition (NTACT). (2015). *Predictor implementation school/district self-assessment*. Retrieved from https://www.transitionta.org/system/files/resources/Predictor_Self-Assessment2.0.pdf?file=1&type=node&id=1359&force=

Newman, I., Wagner, M., Knokey, A., Marder, C., Nagle, K., Shaver, D., & Wei, X. (2011). *The post-high school outcomes of young adults with disabilities up to 8 years after high school: A report from the National Longitudinal Transition Study- 2 (NLTS2)*. Washington, DC: Institute of Education Sciences.

Neitzel, J. (2010). Antecedent-based interventions for children and youth with autism spectrum Disorders: Online training module. (Chapel Hill, NC: National Professional Development Center on Autism Spectrum Disorders, FPG Child Development Institute, UNC-Chapel Hill.) In Ohio Center for Autism and Low Incidence (OCALI). *Autism Internet Modules*, www.autisminternet-modules.org. Columbus, OH: OCALI.

Odom, S.L., Brantlinger, E., Gersten, R., Horner, R.H., Thompson, B. & Harris, K. 2005). Research in special education: Scientific methods and evidence-based practices. *Exceptional Children, 71*,(2) 137-148. Retrieved from https://pdfs.semanticscholar.org/6329/7d39c0c7a2503878705359f2743ed-07b4af4.pdf

O'Reilly, M., Sigafoos, Jeff, Lancioni, G., Edrisinha, C., & Andrews, A. (2005). An examination of the effects of a classroom activity schedule on levels of self-injury and engagement for a child with severe autism. *Journal of Autism and Developmental Disorders, 35*(3), 305-311.

Ostrosky, M., Jung, Y., Hemmeter, L., & Thomas, D. (2008). *Helping children understand routines and classroom schedules* (What Works Brief Series, No. 3). Champaign, IL: University of Illinois at Urbana-Champaign, Center on the Social and Emotional Foundations for Early Learning.

Partin, T.C.M, Robertson, R. E., Maggin, D. M., Oliver, R. M., & Wehby, J. H. (2010). Using teacher praise and opportunities to respond to promote appropriate student behavior. *Preventing School Failure, 54*(3), 172-178.

Patall, Erika & Cooper, Harris & Civey Robinson, Jorgianne. (2008). The Effects of Choice on Intrinsic Motivation and Related Outcomes: A Meta-Analysis of Research Findings. *Psychological Bulletin.* 134. 270-300. 10.1037/0033-2909.134.2.270.

Perry, N. (2009). *Adults on the autism spectrum leave the nest.* London, UK: Jessica Kingsley Publishers.

Pinkelman, S. E., and Horner, R. H. (2017). Improving implementation of function-based interventions: Self-monitoring, data collection, and data review. *Journal of Positive Behavior Interventions, 19*(4), 228-238.

Pratt, C. (2014). Teaching a different way of behaving: Positive behavior supports. In K. D. Buron & P. Wolfberg (Eds.), *Learners on the autism spectrum: Preparing highly qualified educators and related practitioners* (2nd ed., pp. 264-287). Shawnee Mission, KS: AAPC Publishing.

Riffel, L. A., Wehmeyer, M. L., Turnbull, A. P., Lattimore, J., Davies, D., Stock, S., & Fisher, S. (2005). Promoting independent performance of transition-related tasks using a palmtop PC-based self-directed visual and auditory prompting system. *Journal of Special Education Technology, 20,* 5-14.

Rogers, J., & Short, J. (2010). Sensory differences: Online training module (Columbus, OH: Ohio Center for Autism and Low Incidence). In Ohio Center for Autism and Low Incidence (OCALI), *Autism Internet Modules,* www.autisminternetmodules.org. Columbus, OH: OCALI.

Roux, A. M., Rast, J. E., Anderson, K. A., & Shattuck, P. T. (2017). *National autism indicators report: developmental disability services and outcomes in adulthood.* Philadelphia, PA: Drexel University, A. J. Drexel Autism Institute, Life Course Outcomes Research Program.

Roux, A. M., Shattuck, P. T., Rast, J. E., Rava, J. A., & Anderson K. A. (2015). *National autism indicators report: Transition into young adulthood.* Philadelphia, PA: Drexel University, A. J. Drexel Autism Institute, Life Course Outcomes Research Program.

Rutter, M., Maughan, B., Mortimore, P., & Ouston, J. (1979). *Fifteen thousand hours: Secondary schools and their effects on children.* London: Open Books.

Sam, A., & AFIRM Team. (2015). *Visual supports.* Chapel Hill, NC: The University of North Carolina, Frank Porter Graham Child Development Institute, the National Professional Development Center on Autism Spectrum Disorders. Retrieved from http://afirm.fpg.unc.edu/visual-supports

Sam, A., & AFIRM Team. (2016a). *Antecedent-based intervention.* Chapel Hill, NC: The University of North Carolina, Frank Porter Graham Child Development Institute, the National Professional Development Center on Autism Spectrum Disorders. Retrieved from http://afirm.fpg.unc.edu/antecedent-based-intervention

Sam, A., & AFIRM Team. (2016b). *Self-management.* Chapel Hill, NC: The University of North Carolina, Frank Porter Graham Child Development Institute, the National Professional Development Center on Autism Spectrum Disorders. Retrieved from http://afirm.fpg.unc.edu/self-management

Scott, T. M., Alter, P. J., & McQuillan, K. (2010). Functional behavior assessment in classroom settings: Scaling down to scale up. *Intervention in School and Clinic, 46*(2), 87-94.

Shogren, K.A., Faggella-Luby, M.N., Bae, S.J., & Wehmeyer, M.L. (2004). The effect of choice-making as an intervention for problem behavior: A meta-analysis. *Journal of Positive Behavior Interventions 6*(4), 228-237.

Shogren, K. A., & Plotner, A. J. (2012). Transition planning for students with intellectual disability, autism, or other disabilities: Data from the National Longitudinal Transition Study-2. *Intellectual and Developmental Disabilities, 50,* 16-30.

Strategic Instruction Model (SIM). (2019). University of Kansas Center for Research on Learning. Retrieved from https://sim.drupal.ku.edu/slant

Simonsen, B., & Fairbanks, S. (n.d.). *What every teacher should know: Evidence-based practices in classroom management.* Storrs, CT: University of Connecticut, The Center for Behavioral Education and Research. Retrieved from http://apbs.org/Archives/Conferences/fourthconference/Files/Simonsen_fairbanks.pdf

Simonsen, B., Fairbanks, S., Briesch, A., Myers, D., & Sugai, G. (2008). Evidence-based practices in classroom management: Considerations for research to practice. *Education and Treatment of Children, 31*(3), 351-380.

Simonsen, B., Freeman, J., Goodman, S., Mitchell, B., Swain-Bradway, J., Flannery, B., Sugai, G., & Putman, B. (2015). *Supporting and responding to behavior: Evidence-based classroom strategies for teachers.* Washington, DC: U.S. Office of Special Education Programs.

Simpson, R. L., & Myles, B. S. (2007). Understanding and responding to the needs of students with autism. In R. L. Simpson & B. S. Myles (Eds.), *Educating children and youth with autism: Strategies for effective practice.* (2nd ed.). Austin: PRO-ED.

Sugai, G., Horner, R.H., Dunlap, G., Hieneman, M., Lewis, T.J., Nelson, C.M., Scott, T., Liaupsin, C., Sailor, W., Turnbull, A.P., Turnbull III, H.R., Wickham, D., Wilcox, B., & Ruef, M. (2000). Applying positive behavior support and functional behavioral assessment in schools. *Journal of Positive Behavior Interventions, 2*(3), 131-143.

Sutherland, K., Copeland, S., & Wehby, J. (2001). Catch them while you can: Monitoring and increasing the use of effective praise. *Beyond Behavior, 11*(1), 46-49. Retrieved from http://www.jstor.org/stable/24011276

Sutherland, K. S., Wehby, J. H., & Copeland, S.R. (2000). Effect of varying rates of behavior specific praise on the on-task behavior of students with EBD. *Journal of Emotional and Behavioral Disorders, 8,* 2-8.

Test, D. W., Fowler, C., & Kohler, P. (2016). *Evidence-based practices and predictors in secondary transition: What we know and what we still need to know.* National Secondary Transition Technical Assistance Center. Retrieved from https://transitionta.org/system/files/epmatrix/matrix_11_02_17.pdf?file=1&type=node&id=1338

Volden, J., & Johnston, J. (1999). Cognitive scripts in autistic children and adolescents. *Journal of Autism and Developmental Disorders, 29*(3), 203-211.

Wehmeyer, M.L. (2005). Self-determination and individuals with severe disabilities: Reexamining meanings and misinterpretations. *Research and Practice in Severe Disabilities, 30,* 113-120.

Wehmeyer, M.L., Shogren, K.A., Zager, D, Smith, E.C., & Simpson, R. (2010. Research-based principles and practices for educating students autism: Self-determination and social interactions. *Education and Training in Autism and Developmental Disabilities 45*(4), 475-486

Wehmeyer, M.L., & Shogren, K. (2008). Self-determination and learners with autism spectrum disorders. In R. Simpson & B. Myles (Eds.), *Educating children and youth with autism: Strategies for effective practice* (2nd Ed.)(pp.433-476). Austin, TX: Pro-Ed Publishers, Inc.

REFERENCES

Whitney, S. (2017). *Executive functioning skills: Cognitive flexibility*. Student Café Blog. Retrieved from http://blog.studentcaffe.com/cognitive-flexibility/

Wilkins, S., & Burmeister, C. (2015). *FLIPP the switch: Strengthen executive function skills*. Shawnee Mission, KS: AAPC Publishing.

Wong, C., Odom, S. L., Hume, K., Cox, A. W., Fettig, A., Kucharczyk, S., & Schultz, T. R. (2014). *Evidence-based practiced for children, youth, and young adults with Autism Spectrum Disorder*. Chapel Hill, NC: The University of North Carolina, Frank Porter Graham Child Development Institute, Autism-based Review Group.

Wragge, A. (2011). Social narratives: Online training module (Columbus, OH: OCALI). In Ohio Center for Autism and Low Incidence (OCALI). *Autism Internet Modules*, www.autisminternetmodules.org. Columbus, OH: OCALI.

APPENDICES

Appendix A: Chapter 2

Making Changes Student Question Card			
Student:	New Place:		
Where is it located?	❏ indoors	❏ outdoors	
What I saw:	❏ no people	❏ 1-2 people	❏ 10+ people
What I heard:	❏ loud noises	❏ background noise	❏ quiet
What I felt:	❏ anxious & stressed	❏ calm & happy	
How long did I stay in this place?	❏ 5 minutes	❏ 10 minutes	❏ 30+ minutes
Was I comfortable?	❏ Yes	❏ No	
Will I go to this place again?	❏ Yes	❏ No	

Figure 2.6. Making changes individual student question card.

Making Changes Game: Teacher Data Collection Chart				
Student Name:				
Date:	Type of environmental change/name of place:	Length of Time in New Environment *(minutes)*:	Initiated by: S = Student T = Teacher	*MC* Question Card Completed?
		❏ 5 ❏ 10 ❏ 30+	❏ S ❏ T	❏ yes ❏ no
		❏ 5 ❏ 10 ❏ 30+	❏ S ❏ T	❏ yes ❏ no
		❏ 5 ❏ 10 ❏ 30+	❏ S ❏ T	❏ yes ❏ no
		❏ 5 ❏ 10 ❏ 30+	❏ S ❏ T	❏ yes ❏ no

Figure 2.7. Making changes game data collection chart.

Appendix A: Chapter 2

Using Social Narratives Data Collection Chart				
Student Name: _____				
Target Behavior: _____				
Date:	**Situation:**	**Used Narrative?** Y / N	**Target Behavior Exhibited?** Y / N	**Comments:**
		❑ yes ❑ no	❑ yes ❑ no	
		❑ yes ❑ no	❑ yes ❑ no	
		❑ yes ❑ no	❑ yes ❑ no	
		❑ yes ❑ no	❑ yes ❑ no	
		❑ yes ❑ no	❑ yes ❑ no	

Figure 2.11. Social narrative data collection tool.

SOS Strategy Data Collection			
Date	**Student Name**	**Describe Environmental Challenge:** Location/Sensory Impact	**Prompts Needed:** I = Indirect D = Direct N = None
			❑ I ❑ D ❑ N
			❑ I ❑ D ❑ N
			❑ I ❑ D ❑ N
			❑ I ❑ D ❑ N
			❑ I ❑ D ❑ N

Figure 2.14. Class SOS data collection chart.

Appendix A: Chapter 2

Classroom Environment Checklist			
Teacher Name: _____ Date: _____			
❑ Pre-assessment ❑ Post-assessment			
Environmental Component	**Yes**	**No**	**Partial**
1. Individualization and personal connection: Students are given ways to build ownership and a personal connection to the classroom through a display of personal work and interests. Notes: _____			
2. Adaptability and flexibility: The classroom design is flexible enough to allow a variety of activities *or* the design can be changed easily to accommodate different activities. Notes: _____			
3. Color and contrast: The classroom has a good balance of color and is neither too colorful nor too bland. Notes: _____			
4. Visual stimulation: The classroom offers some visual stimulation, but it is not overwhelming. No more than 80% of the wall space is covered. Notes: _____			
5. Lighting: The classroom is well lit and uses primarily natural light, augmented by electric light. If fluorescent light is primarily used, there are areas in the classroom lit by alternate means. Notes: _____			
6. Air quality: There is appropriate circulation of air in the room. Notes: _____			
7. Temperature: The temperature is neither too warm nor too cold. Notes: _____			
8. Use of space and organization: The classroom is well organized and uncluttered. The teacher is able to monitor all areas of the room. Notes: _____			
9. Sound: Classroom noise is minimized through the use of carpet or padded bottoms on chairs and tables. There is no discernable noise from the air conditioner or lighting. Notes: _____			
10. Safe place: There is a safe place available for students to access. This space is designed to provide a sensory break and has fidgets and other items available. Notes: _____			
Totals			

Figure 2.15. Classroom environmental preference checklist.

Appendix A: Chapter 2

Student Environmental Preference Checklist			
Student Name: _____ Date: _____			
Data collector: _____ Role: _____			
☐ Pre-assessment ☐ Post-assessment			
Environmental Component	**Yes**	**No**	**Partial**
1. Color and contrast: Colors are neither too bright nor too dull, and are nice to look at. Notes: _____			
2. Visual stimulation: The walls in the classroom are not too crowded with stuff. Notes: _____			
3. Lighting: The lights in the classroom do not bother me. They are not too bright or too noisy. Notes: _____			
4. Air quality: The room smells OK and is not too stuffy. Notes: _____			
5. Temperature: The temperature isn't too warm or too cold. Notes: _____			
6. Use of space and organization: The classroom looks organized and neat. Notes: _____			
7. Noise Level: The classroom is usually quiet, and there are no noises that bother me. Notes: _____			
Totals			

Figure 2.16. Student environmental preference checklist.

Appendix A: Chapter 2

PLACE Environmental Problem-Solving Chart				
Student:		Teacher:		Date:
Problem	**Let it go?**	**Actions**	**Choose**	**Evaluate**

Figure 2.19. PLACE environmental problem-solving chart used by student and/or teacher.

PLACE Teacher Data Collection				
Student:		Teacher:		Date:
Student completed each step: Independently = I or with Prompts = P				
Problem	**Let it go?**	**Actions**	**Choose**	**Evaluate**
❏ I ❏ P **Comments:**	❏ I ❏ P **Comments:**	❏ I ❏ P **Comments:**	❏ I ❏ P **Comments:**	❏ I ❏ P **Comments:**

Figure 2.20. PLACE teacher data collection tool.

Appendix B: Chapter 3

Task Checklist Time Progress Monitoring		
Name:	Date:	
List the time and tasks or activities to be completed. Did the student complete the task or activity on time? Check yes or no.		
Time to Complete	**Activity**	**Completed on Time?**
		❑Yes ❑ No
		❑Yes ❑ No
		❑Yes ❑ No
		❑Yes ❑ No
		❑Yes ❑ No

Figure 3.2. Task checklist time progress monitoring data collection form.

Visual Schedules Progress Monitoring Form										
Student Name:										
Indicate schedule details based on the Visual Assessment Tool:										
Form of schedule representation (pictures, symbols, words):										
Length of schedule (half day, full day):										
Places schedule will be used (school, home, work):										
Type of schedule (wall, folder, checklist, device):										
Behavior	Date:	Date:	Date:	Date:	Date:	Date:	Date:	Date:	Date:	Date:
1. Initiates using schedule										
2. Follows schedule sequence										
3. Transitions to correct task/area										
4. Accepts changes with no advance warning										
Performance Key: I = Independent P = Prompt O = No Response										
Notes:										

Figure 3.12. Visual schedules progress monitoring form.

Appendix B: Chapter 3

Individual Student Routine Data Collection Worksheet									
Student:				**Routine:**					
Directions: 1. Task analyze routine with steps in first column. 2. Collect baseline data in Column A. 3. Show video daily and practice routine for 1 week; collect 3 data points in B Columns. 4. During weeks 2 -4 collect data 1 time, and enter data in C columns. 5. If scores fall below "8" in Column C, show video and practice routine.							**Scoring Key:** 2 = Independent 1 = Prompt Needed 0 = No Response		
Individual Steps: Date:		**A.**	**B.**	**B.**	**B.**	**C.**	**C.**	**C.**	
1.									
2.									
3.									
4.									
5.									
Mastery = 8 out of 10 points. Total:									
Comments:									

Figure 3.16. Individual routine data collection worksheet

Group Routine Data Collection Worksheet

# Students in Group:		Routine:

Directions:

1. Task analyze routine with steps in first column.
2. Collect baseline data in Column A, counting the number of students who perform the step independently.
3. Show video daily and practice routine for 1 week; collect 3 data points in B Columns by counting students as in Step 2.
4. During weeks 2 -4 collect data 1 time and enter data in C columns by counting students who perform the step independently.
5. Check data in each column. If scores fall below "80%" show video and practice routine.
6. Use the "Individual Student Routine Data Collection" for students who consistently struggle to perform the routine independently.

Scoring Key:

Count and record number of students who complete the step independently.

Individual Steps: Date:	A.	B.	B.	B.	C.	C.	C.
1.							
2.							
3.							
4.							
5.							
Mastery = 80%. **Total:**							

Comments:

Figure 3.17. Group routine data collection worksheet

Appendix B: Chapter 3

MAP: Managing Assignments and Projects Graphic Organizer		
Student Name:		
1. Identify the project assignment and final due date.		
2. Brainstorm the steps needed to complete the assignment. Use a calendar to find due dates for each step.		
3. Write each action step on a sticky note, with the due date in the top corner.		
4. Place each sticky note on your MAP GO in the left column, starting at the top with steps that **need** to get done **first**.		
5. Move tasks that are started, and in progress, to the middle column of the MAP GO.		
6. As each task is completed, move it to the last column on the right side of the MAP GO. *Your goal is to move each sticky note (step) to the right side of the MAP GO.*		
7. For multiple assignments, repeat steps 1-5 using different colored sticky notes, and add to your MAP GO as a visual reminder of the tasks and due dates.		
Not Yet Started	**In Progress**	**Finished**

Figure 3.19. MAP graphic organizer.

Appendix B: Chapter 3

MAP Data Collection				
Start Date	Student Name	Name of Assignment or Project	Number of Assignment/ Project Steps	Number of Steps Completed by Due Dates

Figure 3.20. MAP data collection form.

Figure 3.21. Get it done card template.

Appendix B: Chapter 3

Steps	Get It Done Chart
D-Do it	
O-Options	
N-Needs	
E-Evaluate	

Figure 3.26. Get it done chart.

Get It Done Data Collection Tool				
Date	Student Name	Assignment/ Project Name	What Strategy Was Used	Assignment/ Project Completed
				❑ yes ❑ no
				❑ yes ❑ no
				❑ yes ❑ no
				❑ yes ❑ no

Figure 3.27. Get it done data collection tool.

Appendix B: Chapter 3

Guide for Developing and Teaching Individualized Visual Schedules

Consider the following components when developing and implementing individualized visual schedules:

Schedule Format. Individual visual schedules can take a variety of formats. Representation of information may include photographs, computer program-generated icons, line drawings, written text, or a combination of these. Format examples include:

- a wall schedule with picture/icon cards that the student manipulates (see Figure 3.5),
- a combination picture/word schedule on a clipboard (see Figure 3.6),
- a wipe-off word list on a whiteboard,
- a calendar in a reminder binder (see Figure 3.7),
- paper-pencil check-off lists in notebooks, and
- electronic calendar/scheduling devices.

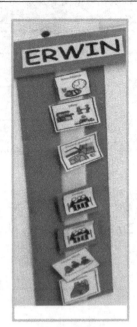

Figure 3.5. Wall Schedule. Communication Symbols ©1981-2015 by Mayer-Johnson LLC a Tobii Dynavox company. All Rights Reserved Worldwide. Used with permission. Boardmaker®is a trademark of Mayer-Johnson LLC.

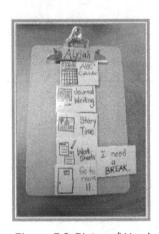

Figure 3.6. Picture/Word

The schedule format is based on the student's strengths and needs. As using special interests can be a powerful way to motivate a student to engage in a desirable behavior (Gagnon & Myles, 2016), a student's highly focused interest may be incorporated into his schedule.

Schedule Length. Consider the length of the schedule. Depending on how successful a student is when presented with the information in his schedule, the individual schedule may be broken into several parts, such as one or two activities, partial day, half day, or full day. For a student whose anxiety level is high when presented with several items on his schedule, a student who is not able to sequence information, or a student with significant attentional difficulties, presenting one item at a time may be effective, with additional items added to the student's schedule as he becomes more successful at independently moving throughout his day.

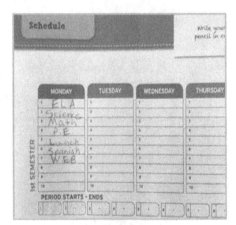

Figure 3.7. Sample of calendar/reminder binder.

Appendix B: Chapter 3

Guide for Developing and Teaching Individualized Visual Schedules *(Continued)*

Student Support. Determine how the student will manipulate the schedule materials throughout the day by considering the following needs the student has when transitioning from through the daily schedule of activities:

- Level of distractibility during transitions.
- Teacher support such as bringing the schedule to him and guiding to the activity.
- Tactile support such as carrying an object/card to match to an identical object/card.
- Marking each schedule change, such as using a check-off system (e.g., Initially, the student may mark off the entire line, then fade to checkmarks).

Schedule Location. Select the appropriate location for the schedule. Schedules can be used in all school environments, including special education classrooms, therapy settings, and general education classes. The schedule should be easy to access but also in a place that will not disturb other students. Following are ways to increasing student independence by providing the appropriate access to their schedule:

- When first using a schedule, staff may move it near the student during transitions.
- As students become more capable, schedules may be located in a central location in a classroom, such the top of a book case or on a wall, where students access their schedule information.
- As students become more independent in using their schedules, they may determine on their own when to check their schedules throughout the day.

Assessing for Student Schedule Needs. The Visual Schedule Assessment Tool (see below) may be used to collect information to determine which type of schedule is most effective for a given student. The important thing to remember is that the individual visual schedule is unique to each student.

As the student makes progress in using uses his schedule, modify the schedule by increasing the level of complexity. For example, for a student who successfully uses a half day schedule, consider transitioning to a full day schedule. For a student who successfully uses a combination picture/word schedule, consider using a written schedule.

Appendix B: Chapter 3

Guide for Developing and Teaching Individualized Visual Schedules *(Continued)*
Visual Schedule Assessment Tool

Name: **Age:**

Directions: *Check the box next to the item in each section that will best meet the needs of the student. Summarize the information to determine the type of schedule that will provide effective visual support for the student.*

Reading Recognition: ❑ Identifies pictures of objects/places ❑ Identifies line drawings/icons ❑ Identifies/reads words of objects/places	Consider the student's ability to recognize and read photos/pictures, icons, and words. The form of representation, needs to match the student's reading level.
Duration or Length of Schedule: ❑ Partial day ❑ Half day ❑ Full day	Duration refers to the number of items shown on the schedule at one time. The schedule may be broken into several parts (i.e., 1 hour, 2 hours, half, full-day).
Where Schedule will Be Used: ❑ In special education classes ❑ In general education classes ❑ On campus or community environments ❑ At home	Consider all environments the student will be in through the school day to determine the type of schedule that will be the most practical.
Type of Schedule to Best Meet Student Needs: ❑ 3x3 cards on a wall strip ❑ 2x2 cards in folder ❑ Picture/word strip in wallet ❑ Wipe-off word list on clipboard ❑ Check-off word list in binder ❑ Electronic device (e.g., smart phone, tablet, etc.)	Based on the student's abilities and needs and the typical environments where the schedule will be used, determine the most appropriate type of schedule for a given student.
Developed by Ruth Prystash & Rebecca Silva, Riverside County Office of Education.	

Appendix C: Chapter 4

Individual Plan For Visual Learning Supports- Elementary	
Directions: Consider how you can increase engagement of your student by providing visual structure to tasks, routines, and activities. This could be in the form of minimal visual supports, or, for students needing more support, task boxes or file folder activities. Is there a way to incorporate student's interest? Use this form to record your ideas.	
Student: Date:	
Type of Task	**How Can I Incorporate Elements of Structure?**

Figure 4.9. Individual plan for visual learning supports form—elementary.

Individual Plan For Visual Learning Supports- Secondary	
Directions: Consider how you can increase engagement of your student by providing visual structure to tasks, routines, and activities. This could be in the form of minimal visual supports, or for students needing more support, task boxes or file folder activities. Is there a way to incorporate student's interest? Use this form to record your ideas.	
Student: Date:	
Type of Task	**How Can I Incorporate Elements of Structure?**

Figure 4.10. Individual plan for visual learning supports form—secondary.

Make a Choice

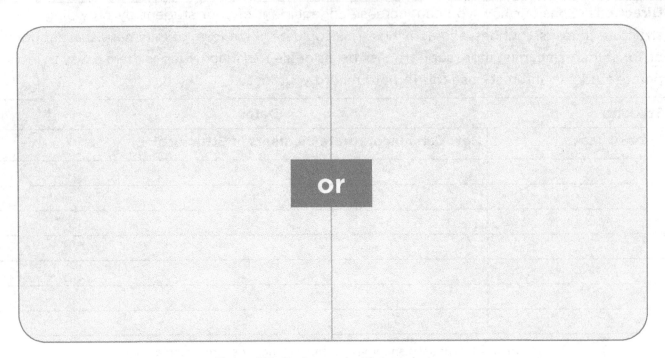

Figure 4.12. Choice card with two choices.

Choice Circle

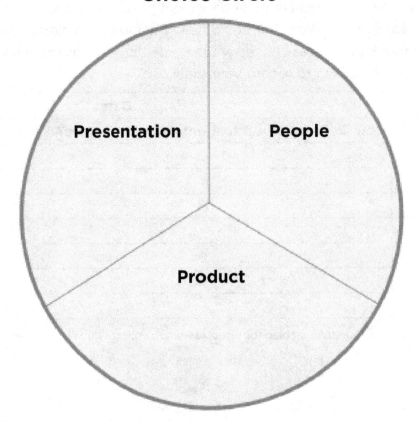

Figure 4.13. Choice circle.

Appendix C: Chapter 4

Choice-Making: Data Collection					
Student Name:					
Date	**Assignment or Project**	**Presentation Choice**	**People Choice**	**Product Choice**	**Assignment Completed**
					❑ yes ❑ no
					❑ yes ❑ no
					❑ yes ❑ no
					❑ yes ❑ no
					❑ yes ❑ no

Figure 4.14. Choice-making data collection tool.

Discussion Cognitive Script: Data Collection					
Student:					
Date:	**Student was prepared:**	**Student met Discussion Expectations:**	**Student Asked Questions:**	**Student Strengths During Discussion:**	**Something Student can work on—next steps:**
	❑ yes ❑ no	❑ yes ❑ no	❑ yes ❑ no		
	❑ yes ❑ no	❑ yes ❑ no	❑ yes ❑ no		
	❑ yes ❑ no	❑ yes ❑ no	❑ yes ❑ no		
	❑ yes ❑ no	❑ yes ❑ no	❑ yes ❑ no		

Figure 4.16. Discussion cognitive script data collection.

Appendix C: Chapter 4

Personal Data Collection Sheet for Discussions		
Student: _____ **Date:** _____		
Place: _____		
1. **Was I prepared?**	☐ Yes ☐ Mostly ☐ Not really	
2. **Did I follow discussion expectations?** *(Yes or No)*		I was respectful
		I listened to others
		I waited for others to finish before speaking
		I stayed on topic
3. **Did I ask questions?** *(Yes or No)*		I asked questions to check my understanding
		I linked my ideas to other people's comments
4. **Things that went well:**		
5. **Things I can work on:**		

Figure 4.17. Personal data collection sheet for discussions.

SLANT Student Data Chart					
Name: ⇨ Write the date. ⇨ Use the key for all five statements. ⇨ In the last row, show how many times you used SLANT for 3-5 minutes in class by making a hash mark each time.			**Key:** Y = Yes N = No S = Sometimes		
Date:					
1. The teacher looked at me more when I used SLANT.					
2. The teacher was more positive when I used SLANT.					
3. I learned more information when I used SLANT.					
4. I took better notes when I used SLANT.					
5. The information was more interesting when I used SLANT.					
Number of times I used SLANT ⇨ 1 mark for every 3-5 minutes that I used SLANT in a fifteen-minute lesson.					

Figure 4.19. SLANT strategy student data chart.

Appendix C: Chapter 4

My Personal Work System Template		
Name:	Location:	Date:
What is the Task?	**What Materials Do I Need?**	
What Do I Do When I'm Finished?		

Figure 4.24. My personal work system template.

Independent Work Progress Monitoring Form					
Student:		Work System Format:		Date:	
Place a number in the column designating the level of independence during work sessions.					
Scoring Key: 2 = Independent, **1** = Prompt needed, **0** = No Response					
	Accesses materials	**Completes task**	**Places work in finished location**	**Transitions to next activity**	**Comments**
Initial Task					
Next Task					
Next Task					
Next Task					
Activity when done		**Comments:**			

Figure 4.25. Independent work progress monitoring form.

Appendix C: Chapter 4

Problem Solving Chart

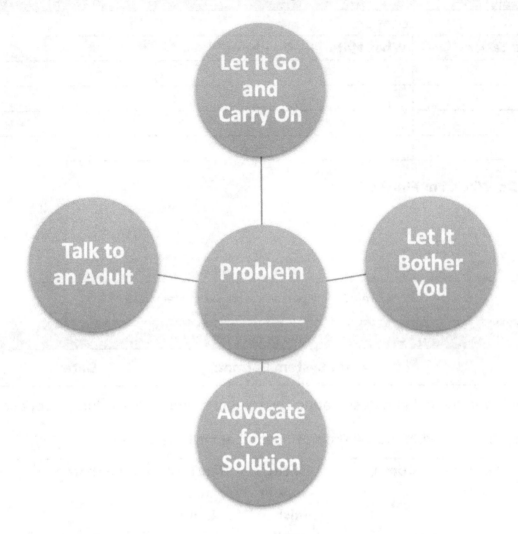

Figure 4.26. Problem-solving chart (Mataya & Owens, 2013). Used with permission.

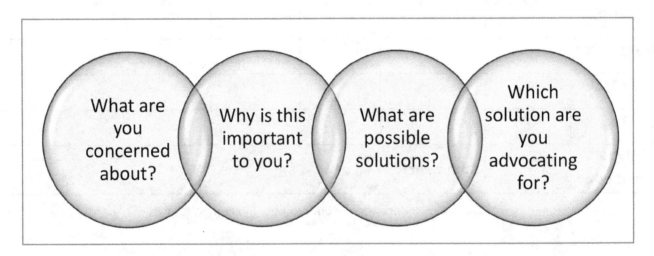

Figure 4.27. 4W Map.

Appendix C: Chapter 4

Self-Advocacy Data Collection			
Student:			
Directions: For each problem listed, describe whether the student used self-advocacy skills and, if so, whether the student initiated the use of the skills or needed a direct or indirect prompt.			
Date	**Describe the Problem**	**Used Self-Advocacy Skills: Y/N**	**Student was:** **I = independent** **P = prompted**
		❏ yes ❏ no	❏ I ❏ P
		❏ yes ❏ no	❏ I ❏ P
		❏ yes ❏ no	❏ I ❏ P
		❏ yes ❏ no	❏ I ❏ P
		❏ yes ❏ no	❏ I ❏ P

Figure 4.28. Self-advocacy data collection tool.

Appendix D: Chapter 5

Quick Function-of-Behavior Questionnaire			
Directions: Answer the following questions regarding a specific behavior of concern. If there are more behaviors that are problematic, choose one to focus on first, and then move on to others.			
Student Name:		**Date:**	
Individual Completing Questionnaire:		**Role:**	
Part One			
1. **What is the problem behavior?** (Describe the behavior as clearly as possible, so that someone not familiar with the student could understand the problem.)			
2. **How often does the behavior occur?**	❑ Hourly ❑ Daily ❑ Weekly ❑ Less often		
3. **How severe is the behavior when it occurs?**	❑ Very severe/dangerous (*If behavior is significant and poses a safety threat to the student or others, an FBA needs to be completed by a behavior specialist.*) ❑ Moderate/some property damage or interruption ❑ Mildly disruptive		
4. **Are there certain settings in which the behavior is *least* likely to occur?**	Days/Times:		
	Activities:		
	People present:		
5. **Are there certain settings in which the behavior is *most* likely to occur?**	Days/Times:		
	Activities:		
	People present:		
6. **What is usually happening to the student prior to the behavior occurring (antecedent)?**			
7. **What usually happens to the student following the behavior occurring (consequence)?**			

Figure 5.3. Function-of-behavior questionnaire–page 1.

Appendix D: Chapter 5

Quick Function-of-Behavior Questionnaire Part Two					
Directions: Rate each item by checking the column that describes the behavior with the following rubric: 5 = Always 4 = Frequently 3 = Sometimes 2 = Not often 1= Never					
Does the problem behavior often occur when the student:	**5**	**4**	**3**	**2**	**1**
1. Is denied access to a preferred activity or object? (A/T)					
2. Is required to participate in a specific activity? (E/T)					
3. Is not receiving attention from peers or adults? (A/A)					
4. Is receiving attention from adults? (E/A)					
5. Does not have access to sensory stimulating activities? (A/S)					
6. Is in an environment with a great deal of sensory input? (E/S)					
Following the problem behavior does the student:	**5**	**4**	**3**	**2**	**1**
7. Receive access to a preferred activity or object? (A/T)					
8. Avoid having to participate in an activity? (E/T)					
9. Get attention (positive/negative) from peers or adults? (A/A)					
10. Avoid attention (positive/negative) from peers/adults? (E/A)					
11. Gain access to sensory stimulating activities? (A/S)					
12. Escape an environment with high sensory input? (E/S)					

Scoring: Add the scores for each function (e.g., A/T, A/A, A/s etc.) using the column values and then write the totals below:			
A/T (Access tangible object/activity) =		E/T (Escape activity) =	
A/A (Access peer/adult attention) =		E/A (Escape peer/adult attention) =	
A/S (Access sensory input) =		E/S (Escape sensory input) =	

Analyze Function of Behavior: If two or more functions score 8 or above, choose one and develop a *Current Behavior Profile* (Table 5.7), *Desired Behavior Profile* (Table 5.8), and *Acceptable Alternative Behavior Profile* (Table 5.11). Collect baseline and intervention data using the *ABC Behavior Data Collection Tool* (Figure 5.4).

Figure 5.3. Function-of-behavior questionnaire–page 2.

Appendix D: Chapter 5

ABC Behavior Data Collection Tool	
Antecedent	
Behavior	
Consequence	

Table 5.4. ABC behavior data collection tool.

Behavior Profile Hypothesis Statement		
Student Name:		
Antecedent	*Behavior*	*Consequence*

Table 5.6. ABC analysis hypothesis statement.

Current Behavior Profile		
Student Name:		
Antecedent	*Behavior*	*Consequence*

Table 5.9. ABC analysis for current behavior.

Appendix D: Chapter 5

Desired Behavior Profile		
Student Name:		
Antecedent	*Behavior*	*Consequence*

Table 5.10. ABC analysis for current behavior.

Acceptable Alternative Behavior Profile		
Student Name:		
Antecedent	**Functionally Equivalent Behavior Strategies**	**Consequence**

Table 5.11. ABC analysis for functionally equivalent behavior strategies.

Appendix D: Chapter 5

Behavior Data Collection Tool				
Student Name: _____				
Person Collecting Data: _____				
Type of data being collected: _____ Baseline _____Intervention				
Collect data for at least **three days** to determine patterns over time. Collect *frequency* data for behaviors that happen often throughout the day but don't last for a long time. Collect *duration* data for behaviors that don't happen often but tend to last for a long time.				
Target behavior (describe the specific behavior in clear terms):				
Date:	**Starting Time:**	**Ending Time:**	**Frequency:**	**Duration:**
Frequency: number of times behavior occurred. Duration: how long behavior occurred.				

Figure 5.4. Behavior data collection tool.

Keep TABS on Your Behavior				
When	**Where**	**What**	**Duration/Frequency**	**Reentry Plan**

Figure 5.11. Blank TABS worksheet.

Data Collection: TABS (Take a Break Strategy)				
Name:				
Date/Time	**Activity**	**Location**	**Break Initiated by**	**Duration**

Figure 5.12. Data collection tool for TABS.

Appendix D: Chapter 5

Teacher Self-Monitoring of Positive to Negative Statements					
Teacher Name:			**Data collected by:**		
Directions: Count the number of times you make positive statements (statements praising a student or group of students) and negative statements (ones that are corrective).					
Date	**Time**	**Lesson/Activity**	**# Positive**	**# Negative**	**Ratio of positive/ negative**

Figure 5.13. Data-collection tool for positive vs. negative feedback ratio.

Precorrection Data Collection							
Student name:							
Setting:							
Potential problems:							
Supports identified:							
Date	**Supports Used**	**Independently Used Supports**			**Student Feedback**		
		Yes	**No**	**Partial**	**Positive**	**Negative**	**Neutral**

Figure 5.15. Precorrection data collection chart.

Appendix E: Chapter 6

Predictors/Outcomes	Education	Employment	Independent Living
Career Awareness – learning about opportunities, education, and skills needed	X	X	
Community Experiences – activities outside of school supported with in-class instruction		X	
Exit Exam Requirements/HS – standardized state tests students must pass to receive a diploma		X	
Goal Setting – vocational goal setting through student participation in the IEP	X	X	
Inclusion in General Education – access to general ed. curriculum and peers	X	X	X
Interagency Collaboration – cross-agency, program, and disciplinary collaboration	X	X	
Occupational Courses – support of career awareness, exploration, and experiences	X	X	
Paid Employment/Work Experience – job shadowing, internships, competitive employment	X	X	X
Parent Expectations – support and encouragement of high parent expectations related to specific desired outcomes	X	X	X
Parental involvement – support and encouragement of active parent involvement in transition planning		X	
Program of Study – courses, experiences, and curriculum to support post-school goals		X	
Self-Care/Independent Living Skills – personal care, daily living skills, financial, and health care	X	X	
Self-Advocacy/Self-Determination – making choices, solving problems, setting goals, accepting consequences of actions	X	X	X
Social Skills – behaviors, actions, attitudes promoting communication and cooperation	X	X	
Student Support – support network that helps with resources to attain transition goals	X	X	X
Transition Program – preparing students to plan and move from school to adult life	X	X	
Travel Skills – training students to travel independently outside the home to increase employment success		X	
Vocational Education – courses that prepare students for a specific job or career	X	X	
Work Study – work experiences on or off campus earning high school credit		X	
Youth Autonomy/Decision Making – opportunities for students to make everyday decisions (e.g., plan school activities, both short and long-range)	X	X	

Table 6.2. Predictors of successful secondary transition learning strategies for future.
From: https://transitionta.org/system/files/effectivepractices/EBPP_Exec_Summary_2016_12_13_16.pdf

Appendix E: Chapter 6

What's My PLAN?	
PLAN	**Answers and Solutions**
P = Is there a <u>P</u>roblem?	
L = Is it <u>L</u>ittle or Big?	
A = Plan <u>A</u> and Plan B?	
N = <u>N</u>ext step?	

Figure 6.3. What's my PLAN chart for problem solving.

PLAN Data Collection			
Student: _____			
Directions: For each problem listed, describe whether the student used the PLAN Steps and, if so, whether the problem was solved.			
Date	**Describe the Problem**	**Used PLAN Steps Y/N**	**Problem Solved Y/N**
		❑ yes ❑ no	❑ yes ❑ no
		❑ yes ❑ no	❑ yes ❑ no
		❑ yes ❑ no	❑ yes ❑ no
		❑ yes ❑ no	❑ yes ❑ no
		❑ yes ❑ no	❑ yes ❑ no

Figure 6.4. PLAN strategy data collection tool.

Appendix E: Chapter 6

Visual Scale Data Collection					
Level of Emotion: *(See the 5-Point Scale)*	**5 Extremely Anxious** 😢 Take break and ask for help	**4 Really Anxious** 😟 Take short walk	**3 Anxious** 😐 Use deep breathing app	**2 Calm to Anxious** 😐 Take action and I'll be OK	**1 Calm & OK** 😊 Keep doing what I'm doing

Name:		**Place:**	❑ Home	❑ School	❑ Work

Directions: Pick one place (home, school, work) and keep track of your emotions for five days by using your *Visual Scale*.

Date:	My level of emotion was: _____	I used the Visual Scale: ❑ yes ❑ no	I reduced my anxiety: ❑ yes ❑ no	If no, what will I do next time:
Date:	My level of emotion was: _____	I used the Visual Scale: ❑ yes ❑ no	I reduced my anxiety: ❑ yes ❑ no	If no, what will I do next time:
Date:	My level of emotion was: _____	I used the Visual Scale: ❑ yes ❑ no	I reduced my anxiety: ❑ yes ❑ no	If no, what will I do next time:
Date:	My level of emotion was: _____	I used the Visual Scale: ❑ yes ❑ no	I reduced my anxiety: ❑ yes ❑ no	If no, what will I do next time:
Date:	My level of emotion was: _____	I used the Visual Scale: ❑ yes ❑ no	I reduced my anxiety: ❑ yes ❑ no	If no, what will I do next time:

Figure 6.6. Visual scale data collection tool for students.

Appendix E: Chapter 6

Interview Data Collection Worksheet						
Student:						
Directions: • Write the name of the interviewer. • Write the date of the interview. • Score yourself on each of the six behaviors. • Add up your scores. • Continue to practice skills with scores of 1 and 0 points.				**Scoring Key:** Yes-Did it well = 2 OK-Sometimes = 1 No-Not at all = 0		
Interviewer:	Date:	Date:	Date:	Date:	Date:	
1. Greeted the Interviewer: made eye contact, shook hands, said hello.						
2. Looked at and listened to the interviewer.						
3. Asked questions when I didn't understand something.						
4. Answered each question to the best of my ability.						
5. Looked at the interviewer and gave eye contact a few times during my answers.						
6. Said "thank you" at the end of the interview.						
Mastery = 10 -12 points. **Total:**						
Comments:						

Figure 6.8. Interview data collection tool for students.

Appendix E: Chapter 6

Networking Worksheet			
Name:	**Date:**		
Make a Network List • *Names of Family & Friends* • *Phone Numbers* • *Ask for job contacts*	**Name** _____ _____ _____		**Phone Number** _____ _____ _____
List Job Lead Contacts • *Names of Contact & Company* • *Phone Numbers*	**Contact Name & Company** _____ _____ _____		**Phone Number** _____ _____ _____
	Company A	**Company B**	**Company C**
Select Three Companies & Jobs to Research • Company facts • What they do • Jobs you would like			
List Questions to Ask About- • *Job openings* • *Requirements for jobs–education and experience* • *Advice for a potential job candidate*			
Call the Contact • Write date of call			
Send Thank You • Write date sent			
Prepare to Answer Questions	*Review your Career Search Portfolio* and have it in front of you when you make the call. When you are asked questions, you can refer to information in the portfolio.		

Figure 6.11. Networking worksheet for student job search.

Appendix E: Chapter 6

SOARR Chart				
Specify	**Observe**	**Analyze**	**Respond**	**Reflect**
What is the context or specific situation?	What do I see in this situation? How are other people behaving?	What do I need to do to fit in to this situation? What questions do I need to ask and answer in my head?	Based on my analysis of the situation, what did I do?	What happened? What did I learn? What will I do differently next time?

Figure 6.12. SOARR Chart–blank template.

SOARR Data Collection				
Date	**Student Name**	**Describe the Problem**	**Used SOARR Strategy? Y/N**	**Solved Problem? Y/N**
			❏ yes ❏ no	❏ yes ❏ no
			❏ yes ❏ no	❏ yes ❏ no
			❏ yes ❏ no	❏ yes ❏ no
			❏ yes ❏ no	❏ yes ❏ no
			❏ yes ❏ no	❏ yes ❏ no

Figure 6.13. SOARR class data collection chart.

CPSIA information can be obtained
at www.ICGtesting.com
Printed in the USA
BVHW091924170721
612126BV00016B/1065